This book is to be returned on or before
the last date stamped below.

20. NOV. 1993

103940/1

TAYSIDE COLLEGE OF NURSING AND MIDWIFERY

LIBREX

Community Psychiatric Nursing
myth and reality

Linda C Pollock

BSc, PhD, RGN, Dist Nurs Cert, Dip Clin Nurs (Edin), RMN

Dissertation submitted for the degree of Doctor of
Philosophy from the University of Edinburgh

ROYAL COLLEGE OF NURSING
RESEARCH SERIES

Scutari Press

Aims of the Series
To encourage the appreciation and dissemination of nursing research by making relevant studies of high quality available to the profession at reasonable cost.

The RCN is happy to publish this series of research reports. The projects were chosen by the individual research worker and the findings are those of the researcher and relate to the particular subject in the situation in which it was studied. The RCN in accordance with its policy of promoting research awareness among members of the profession commends this series for study but views expressed do not necessarily reflect RCN policy.

Scutari Press

Viking House, 17–19 Peterborough Road,
Harrow, Middlesex HA1 2AX, England

A subsidiary of Scutari Projects, the publishing company of
the Royal College of Nursing

First published 1989

British Library Cataloguing in Publication Data:

Pollock, Linda
    Community psychiatric nursing
    1. Great Britain. Psychiatric patients.
    Nursing
    I. Title
    610.73'68'0941

    ISBN 1–871364–18–3

Typeset by Action Typesetting Ltd., Gloucester
Printed and bound in Great Britain by Billing & Sons, Worcester

'It is necessary to warn the reader that any appearance of clarity and systemization, which references to this research might give – is largely a retrospective phenomenon. The actual process of arriving at one's aims seems to the writer to be a muddled one! Clarification does not appear to be achieved with a few clever discussions with one's colleagues or by a few final inspirations. It appears rather as an outcome of experience, and a good deal of muddled thought, with the results that one's aims are subjected to frequent modifications. Sometimes one finds that one has been carrying out certain aims before one is aware of them, or that one is doing things which are directly contrary to one's clearest formulations. The only thing one can say with confidence is that the achievement of clarity depends on the ability simultaneously to tolerate two opposite experiences: a realisation that one is in a muddle on certain points, and a determination to get out of it.'

(Shapiro, 1963, quoted in Sainsbury P and Kreitman N (eds.), 'A Clinical Approach to Fundamental Research', Oxford University Press.)

Contents

Preface

'Between the idea and the reality. Between the motion and the act. Falls the shadow' (TS Eliot, 'The Hollow Men.')

Within these covers you will find a wealth of information about several realities:

- *The reality of community psychiatric nursing* – what nurses think they are doing is set against what they are actually doing.
- *The reality of 'community care'* – how the policy and political rhetoric do not square with the resource allocations which ensure an expansion of a range of services to the mentally ill.
- *The reality of consumer feedback* – what the patients and informal carers, as recipients, find helpful about contact with community psychiatric nurses. This gives some useful insights about perceptions of practice which do not necessarily mirror the expressed goals of the nurses.
- *The reality of research* – the documentation of a research study which evaluates nursing practice as complicated and diverse as that of community psychiatric nursing.

You can use the text to tap into one or all of these realities.

This book is a published version of a thesis which was presented for a PhD degree at Edinburgh University in 1987. A volume of the thesis has been placed in the Steinberg Collection of theses, based in the Royal College of Nursing's library in London. The substance of the original thesis remains almost intact. The decision to retain the essence of the thesis was underpinned by two reasons.

Firstly, the work, by its presentation, clearly details the process involved in 'doing' research: reviewing the literature; designing the study (choice and rationale of the methods and tools used); developing a timetable; gaining access to the research areas; surmounting the practicalities imposed by the research setting; conducting the pilot and main studies; and, finally, analysing and presenting the findings. A strength of the work is that the completed study, as it is written, identifies some of the pitfalls of the chosen research methodology. It was considered important to have this depth of detail preserved in order to pass on valuable information to the nurse reader wishing to embark on a research project.

The purpose of a PhD degree is to teach the student an appreciation of research method; thus, the graduate can tackle problems systematically and objectively, and hence find appropriate solutions. A strength of the original thesis is that it presented both a qualitative and a quantitative approach to a research problem; details of methodology are given which could be of practical use to other budding researchers. This was the second reason why almost the entire thesis was published in book form.

The completed study recorded within this text should furnish all workers involved in community care (whatever that means, see chapter 2), with up-to-date and relevant information about community psychiatric nursing. The myth of the provision of 'individualised' care is exploded and the reality of 'juggling resources' revealed. This finding has implications for nursing practice, nurse educationalists and managers, and is noteworthy considering the present political/economic climate. The study also shows details of practice hitherto unknown, in particular, nurses' use of the social model of care, and the fact that nurses succeed in making an under-resourced system work. This, combined with the findings that comprehensive care is not offered to informal carers, and that the latter are seen as secondary to patients, should be urgently noted by planners and politicians.

The issues to be addressed by future community psychiatric nursing services are factors worthy of examination by all those interested in the provision of care for the emotionally distressed. These factors include the organisation of community psychiatric nursing services generally, as well as the organisation of the community psychiatric nurses' work at clinical level.

Because the demands placed on any one service are influenced by the scope and nature of other available services, this topic must be tackled by the range of disciplines involved in planning care for the mentally ill. Other priorities for these planners are to integrate a research component into all new community care developments and to evaluate and monitor the performance of existing services. At the clinical level, high standards of nursing practice can only be ensured along with efficient use of resources if three strategies are considered: first, the integration of clinical supervision into community psychiatric nursing work; second, the incorporation of training and practice to improve skills and teach systematic methods of work; third, a more explicit use of conceptual models. These proposed strategies are focused on in the final chapter.

This book comprises five chapters. At the beginning of chapter 1, the aims and objectives of the study are outlined; this is followed by a review of personal and professional reasons for the study. In the remaining part of chapter 1, the 'conceptual framework' is elaborated; this provides the conceptual basis for the present study and outlines thinking which crucially affected the design of the study. Chapter 2 consists of the literature review. This sets the study into context and examines some of the issues relevant to both community psychiatric nursing and the emergent study. The third chapter details the study itself and focuses on the methodology. Chapter 4 presents and discusses the results. The fifth, and closing, chapter summarises the main issues that arose from the data and underlines some of the wider implications that emerge from the study.

It is impossible to mention by name all the many individuals who in small ways influenced the formation of this work. At the top of this list must be those involved in awarding me a Scottish Home and Health Department Nurse Research Training Fellowship – this award was responsible for the inception and continuation of the study. Also close to the top must be the nurses, patients and carers who took part in the research, without whom this study would not have been possible; all gave considerable time to the demands of the study with a co-operation and willingness which made the data collection phase especially enjoyable. I ask you all simply to accept my gratitude.

I would further like to mention and thank some key individuals without whose enthusiasm and support this book would never have been published: Professor Annie Altschul, Dr Kath Melia, Dr Susan Sladden, Steve Smythe, José Closs, Dr Mike Barfoot, Clodagh Ross and Professor Dave Smythe – I am indebted to each and every one of you.

1 Introduction

AIMS AND OBJECTIVES

Objectives

The main objectives were

1. to find out whether community psychiatric nursing is effective;
2. to develop a research tool to evaluate community psychiatric nursing services.

Primary aims

These objectives were achieved by evaluating two community psychiatric nursing services. This evaluation was, firstly, at the level of individual practice, to provide qualitative information about the 'process' of community nursing, and, secondly, in relation to the patients' and families' response to this service, to provide 'outcome' information.

Process evaluation

It is not clear from the literature what goals community psychiatric nurses are aiming for. The goals for community psychiatric nursing activity tend to have been stated in imprecise, broad terms (see p.42), and the available quantitative measures tell us little about their attainment (see p.61). Some goals of community psychiatric nursing activity can, of course, be measured in quantitative terms, but many others, e.g. improving a patient's social skills or his capacity to cope with stress, are less amenable to quantitative measures. The present research aimed to provide a broad analysis of community psychiatric nursing practice and to examine the values and assumptions underpinning the work of the community psychiatric nurses. The work of community psychiatric nursing specifically with carers was also explored.

1

Outcome evaluation

The 'outcome' part of the study discovered how carers perceive community psychiatric nurses, and how carers' experience of problems is relieved by community psychiatric nursing intervention. The literature on community care approaches in psychiatry suggests that one of the major effects of the change in orientation of care is that patients spend less time in hospital and more time with the people with whom they live. This effect of placing more responsibility on the family is loosely described as 'burden' in the literature. This term, first coined by Grad and Sainsbury (1963, 1968) and elaborated later by Hoenig and Hamilton (1965, 1967, 1969), refers to the hardship that families suffer in adjusting their life-style to accommodate a mentally-ill person. One of the rationales for developing community psychiatric nursing has been to support families and carers of the mentally ill.

The patients' view of community psychiatric nursing was also obtained because it seemed unethical to approach relatives without the permission of the psychiatric patients in the study.

Secondary aims

These were:

1.   to examine practice with a view to highlighting the training needs of community psychiatric nurses;
2.   to examine practice with a view to focusing on organisational factors relevant to community psychiatric nursing;
3.   to review service goals in the community.

These aims were achieved by:

1.   describing and comparing the work of community psychiatric nurses in two different areas. This established a picture of the way in which a small number of community psychiatric nurses worked;
2.   eliciting the families' and patients' views of the two community psychiatric nursing services;
3.   identifying what it is that patients and families find helpful about community psychiatric nursing contact. This permitted an evaluation of the community psychiatric nursing service in terms of the family's perception of their problems as alleviated by the community psychiatric nursing contact.

This research focuses on gaps in current knowledge.

THE BACKGROUND TO THE PRESENT STUDY

This study was motivated by a concern to examine critically the work of community psychiatric nurses. This motivation arose out of doubts

I had about the efficacy of community psychiatric nursing. These became all the more acute when faced with the reality of the practice situation, which gave contradictory and confusing feedback about the work of community psychiatric nursing. Patients, carers and other workers, voluntary and professional, for example, could be either for or against the development of this speciality; there were also conflicting views on the efficacy of community psychiatric nursing within psychiatric nursing itself.

The main reason for my interest was that I had been working in the speciality of community psychiatric nursing for almost five years. This was at a time when psychiatry generally was suffering from shortages of nursing staff. This was a factor commented on by the Scottish Mental Welfare Commission:

> 'The most serious problem facing staff in their task of caring for patients is the shortage of nurses. It has been emphasised that this has ill-effects on the treatment and management of every type of psychiatric patient and that there are also worrying effects on the training and on the morale of the staff themselves.' (Mental Welfare Commission, 1986)

The development of specialities like community psychiatric nursing has compounded the existing shortage of trained psychiatric nurses in hospitals – a concern which the Scottish Hospital Advisory Service has expressed on several occasions:

> 'We are pleased to note the developments of community psychiatric nursing services and day hospitals ... but to some extent this has been at the expense of adequate numbers of trained staff in the long stay and geriatric psychiatry units.' (Scottish Home and Health Department, 1983)

The fact that the speciality of community psychiatric nursing was developing at the expense of hospital-based provision of care presented a major dilemma for me as a practitioner.

On the one hand, I was committed professionally to high standards of care given by nurses in the community setting. I, therefore, maintained a high profile and continually argued for a numerical increase in, and the development of, nurses working in the community setting, in order to cope with the ever-increasing demands made of the limited number of nurses in post. The service managers indicated that an increased availability of nursing staff for community work would result in hospital shortages. Their priority was a responsibility for hospitalised patients whose needs were immediate and visible. This response, reflecting the hospital orientation of the provision of the current psychiatric nursing services, reinforced my resolve to maintain the work of community psychiatric nursing on a high profile.

Attached to an acute admission ward, from which I received two-thirds of referrals, I ensured that hospital-based colleagues were aware of my work as a community psychiatric nurse, and I involved them in decisions about the nature of the work. I was also actively involved in the Community Psychiatric Nurses Association, a professional organisation whose expressed aim is to speak out on issues relevant to community psychiatric nursing.

Sometimes, however, I could not help but question the wisdom of whether scarce resources (i.e. trained psychiatric nurses) should be diluted by the current, although limited, allocation of staff to community work. Should they not be concentrated on the areas of most pressing need, rather than continuing at present with the 'robbing Peter to pay Paul' philosophy which provided a crisis management service? With this query in mind, I was interested in discovering more about the actual effects of community psychiatric nursing. It was perhaps a naive hope, but I anticipated that the findings would provide a solid foundation from which to argue for or against the future provision of community psychiatric nursing.

My work experience suggested that the local development of community psychiatric nursing was dependent on the personal interests of the community psychiatric nurses or the influence of other workers such as nurse managers, GPs or psychiatrists. Planned development of community psychiatric nursing, linked with clear objectives or assessment of whether or not these had been achieved, seemed to be absent. The opportunity to do research afforded the chance to examine the broader picture of community psychiatric nursing and to focus on this issue more objectively.

A second major influence of my 'community' experience on the present research study was that community psychiatric nursing was, at that time, assessed quantitatively, a form of measurement which did not accurately reflect the work of community psychiatric nurses (see p.61). Undertaking the present research study afforded the opportunity to investigate other methods of evaluating community psychiatric nursing. The solitary nature of the job, with an emphasis on unsupervised work in the home-visiting situation, meant that a large part of community psychiatric nursing work was based on individual decision-making. I was interested in discovering more about the actual work of community psychiatric nursing and, in particular, the values and assumptions underpinning the work.

Finally, this study was prompted by two other less personal and more general factors, first, the increased development of community psychiatric nursing epitomised by the attention given to 'community psychiatric nursing' in policy documents, and, second, the current emphasis in health care generally (Donabedian, 1983), and psychiatric nursing in particular, on research and evaluation of services (Wilson-Barnett, 1983; Brooking, 1986). These factors combined to make the present research both timely and relevant.

THE CONCEPTUAL FRAMEWORK

The research question formulated for examination at the outset of the research study was, 'Is community psychiatric nursing effective?' With this in mind, the next section presents some of the literature in the area of health-care evaluation and how it influenced the present study.

Two major influences on the present study can be identified: these are Suchman's model of the intellectual process of evaluation and Donabedian's model of the foci or mind's eye objects of evaluation. The relevance of these is elaborated below.

Initial reading indicated that the word 'effective' focused on the ability of a programme to be carried out successfully. Other words, 'effects' and 'efficiency', continually emerged in the literature in relation to 'evaluation'. The 'effects' of a programme are defined as the ultimate influence of a programme on a target, and 'efficiency' as how well, and at what cost relative to other ways of producing similar effects (Wright, 1955; Cochrane, 1971).

The mere mention of some of the phrases and words – 'ultimate influence', 'successfully', 'relative to other ways', suggested that the task ahead would not be easy! 'Ultimate influence' suggested that activities may have grades of influence. Who judges whether an action is successful or not?; the same activity may be judged as both unsuccessful and successful by different assessors. Suchman (1967, pp.31–2) defined 'evaluation' as:

'... the determination (*whether based on opinions, records, subjective or objective data*) of the results (*whether desirable or undesirable, transient or permanent, immediate or delayed*) attained by some activity (*whether a program, or part of a program, a drug or a therapy, an ongoing or one-shot approach*) designed to accomplish some valued goal or objective (*whether ultimate, intermediate, or immediate, effort or performance, long or short range*). This definition contains four key dimensions: (1) process – the 'determination'; (2) criteria – the 'results'; (3) stimulus – the 'activity'; and (4) value – the 'objective'. The scientific method ... provides the most promising means for 'determining' the relationship of the 'stimulus' to the 'objective' in terms of measurable 'criteria' (my italics).

This definition, although helpful overall, tends to confound values with objectives. Suchman continues:

'The value-laden nature of one's objectives constitutes a major distinction between evaluative research and basic research aimed at hypothesis testing. A precondition to an evaluation study is the presence of some activity whose objectives are assumed to have value.'

Values are generally seen at a higher level of abstraction than are the goals derived from them. According to King (1962), 'Values are the principles by which we establish priorities and hierarchies of

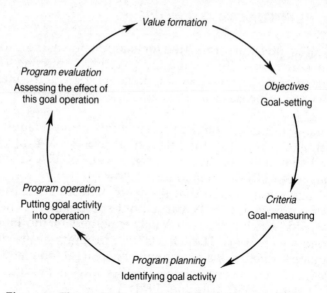

Figure 1 The evaluation process (after Suchman, 1967)

importance among needs, demands, and goals'. In terms of King's definition, values underlie or determine our goals and are thus of a prior and separate order from either goals or objectives. 'Values' of course, are very closely tied to the setting up of goals – one does not ask if something is of value without asking, 'Value for what?'. This is recognised by Suchman (1967) who argues that the evaluation process itself stems from and returns to the formation of values.

Figure 1 shows Suchman's final visualisation of the evaluation process. To take an example from community psychiatric nursing, the value could be 'That the dignity of individuals should be preserved or that all adults have a right to participate in community life'. Arising from this, the goal set could be, 'Admission to psychiatric hospital should be avoided or the number of admissions to psychiatric hospitals should be reduced'. In order to measure whether or not this goal is achieved, statistics on admissions could be obtained. The 'goal-attaining activities' could then be identified, e.g. early sufferers detected, support services developed in the community for patients and families, or domicillary visiting organised. These activities would then be put into operation; liaison with GPs, health visitors and social workers would be organised on a regular basis, premises would be secured for day centres, social clubs or self-help groups which would be advertised locally and via professionals, and practical arrangements made about who would run and organise the group. These goal-directed operations would be assessed to see if the stated predetermined objectives had been achieved. Finally the initial value is reassessed.

This scheme suggests that it is possible to isolate dimensions to be measured. The present study attempted to examine the values, assumptions and goal activities of the community psychiatric nurses and see if these were identifiable and separable.

Separation of the assumptions and goal activities of community psychiatric nurses may not be possible:

'The many difficulties suggested – the breadth of the thing subsumed under a particular objective, the multiple objectives encompassed by many programs, the ambiguity inherent in any or all of the objectives as stated, and the disagreement as to the objectives – are characteristic of many programs and are enough to stagger the imagination of the evaluator.' (Hyman et al, 1962)

Despite the fact that health-care programmes have multiple objectives, three types of 'goal' have been described: immediate, intermediate and ultimate.

'Practically, there can be very little argument about this requirement that immediate and intermediate goals constitute valid steps towards the attainment of some ultimate goal. Otherwise activity becomes substituted for effect and the goals that lead to the adoption of certain means tend to be forgotten as the means become ends in and of themselves. However knowledge is never complete and there must always be gaps in the 'cause/effect' sequence which can only be filled by making assumptions concerning the validity of the intermediate steps ... such linkages are often if not usually taken for granted but upon challenge they must be reproducible. (Suchman, 1967)

The present study aimed to explore and examine the goals of community psychiatric nursing as described by community psychiatric nurses.

The work of Donabedian (1966) offered a framework for health service evaluation focusing on structure, process and outcome. These were examined by Bloch (1975) with particular reference to nursing:

Structure: involves the study of factors of the system such as equipment, physical facilities, staffing levels and patterns, styles of supervision and management and characteristics of the care givers, attitudes and training.
Process: involves the 'process' of giving care, namely what the care giver does. This includes visible behaviour but also invisible actions such as decision making.
Outcome: the results of care are examined in terms of change in the recipient of care.

The above synopsis of evaluation research helped to focus my area of investigation. The literature review shows that there is a dearth of evaluative research on community psychiatric nursing. Studies examining the 'process' of community psychiatric nursing have tended to be quantitative rather than qualitative in nature. These studies focus on numbers (e.g. of case-loads, referrals or visits) and are limited because they do not provide meaningful measurements on which to determine clinical input, safe practice or forward planning. The few 'outcome' studies have been on specialised patient populations. Examination of the 'process' of community psychiatric nursing in this study was qualitative in nature and made explicit the goals and assumptions of the community psychiatric nurses. An 'outcome' evaluation of community psychiatric nursing, by looking at the consumers' view of that care, was also attempted.

2 | Review of the literature

THE CONCEPT OF COMMUNITY CARE
Introduction

Goals at policy level are essential to the context of the service at organisation and practice level. In this section, 'community care' as a policy goal is examined. This draws attention to the ambiguities inherent in the definitions of 'community care'. Consideration of the concept is broadened beyond the administrative structure to focus on care *in*, *for* and *by* the community.

Goals at policy-making level

The term 'community care' is not a contemporary one. Suggestions of moves in that direction can be picked out of the literature. At the turn of the century, the Local Government Board recommended 'more homely' accommodation than the workhouse (Personal Social Services Council/Central Health Services Council, 1978). In 1918, the Board of Control of Mental Hospitals recommended early treatment of acute cases in general hospitals, and the Royal Commission on Lunacy and Mental Disorder (1924–1926) combined with the annual reports of the Board of Control to add pressure for the appointment of almoners (medical social workers) to help keep families together (Lonsdale et al, 1980). It was not until after World War II that the policy of 'community care' became explicit.

'Community care' is a policy uniting politicians, planners, social service and health-care professionals and a wide range of pressure groups. 'Community care' has been a prominent policy goal of governments and a central guiding principle in the development of health and social services of both major political parties since World War II.

Community care definitions

For such a pervasive concept, definition of 'community care' is surprisingly elusive. Sladden (1979), for instance, has commented:

'The phrase community care has become something of a slogan used

9

without precision and in different senses in various contexts . . . The term is indiscriminately used to denote either a principle of administration or the actual range of services provided. Similarly 'the community' is used to denote both a social group and a territory.'

One of the most recent official documents on community care has commented:

'The phrase "community care" means little in itself. It is a phrase used by some descriptively, by others prescriptively: that is by some, as a shorthand way of describing certain specific services provided in certain ways and certain places; by others as an ideal principle in the light of which existing services are to be judged and new ones developed. It has in fact come to have such general reference as to be virtually meaningless.' (Social Services Committee Report, 1985)

The difficulty of 'community care' definitions was acknowledged by the DHSS Report (1981b) which classified these into two types, detailed below. The report draws a distinction between:

'definitions which *describe* the services and resources which are involved (eg community care is those services provided outside of institutions . . .) and those which are in effect *statements of objectives* (eg community care is minimising the disruption of ordinary living . . .). Although it would not seem fruitful to offer one all-purpose definition it is important to specify what is meant whenever the term is used.' (Department of Health and Social Security, 1981b, my italics)

This DHSS report suggested that the switching between the two different uses of the term 'community care' is the cause of confusion. The confusion also results from the inadequacy of the distinctions. The report continues:

'Used *descriptively* community care sometimes means those services provided by local authority social services departments rather than the NHS. This shorthand stems from the main policy thrust, stressed particularly in the late 1960s and early 1970s, of shifting the main responsibility for some people, particularly some long-stay hospital patients, from NHS to the PSS . . . the objectives, explicit or implicit in statements about community care, range from the very specific to all encompassing approaches to care giving. The client group in relation to which objectives are set is perhaps the most important variable. But the nature of the resources available and current practice patterns in a given locality also help fashion objectives.'

This discussion hints at the reality of service provision, which is complicated and cannot be successfully reduced to simple watertight definitions. 'Community (health-) care' services themselves present problems of definition. Primary health-care services include GPs, health visitors and district nurses and deal with some 90% of cases of mental illness (see Goldberg and Huxley, 1980, for a discussion of this figure), yet the GP and community nursing services are funded differently. Personal Social Service staff often exclude residential care when they use the term 'community care'. Frequently, therefore, 'community care' is used to mean all services provided outside institutions, regardless of which agency (NHS, voluntary or Personal Social Services) provides them. This distinction is also problematic – do hostels come under the institutional umbrella? What about community-based packages of care which combine using the institution and other supportive resources, e.g. short spells of planned hospital admission or hospital day-care with community psychiatric nurse follow-up, meals-on-wheels and provision of the home-help service?

A further complication is a growing tendency to equate 'community care' with the support provided by individuals in a given community to its own most vulnerable members, and to exclude formally-provided services, whether from statutory agencies or the organised voluntary sector.

Government policy documents advocating the development of 'community care' do not clarify matters (see Department of Health and Social Security, 1971, 1974, 1975, 1976, 1981a, 1981b; Social Services Committee Report, 1985; Scottish Home and Health Department, 1976, 1979a, 1979b, 1980a, 1980b, 1985). These do not have a clear or consistent definition of the term.

Official reports also present confused aims and suggest ambiguities in outlined policies; this is epitomised most frequently by discussion of 'community care' without an elaboration of proposed strategies. The Department of Health and Social Security (1971), for example, expressed commitment to community care but argued that the services in greatest need of expansion were residential homes; a target of a 15% increase in the number of residental places was set without planning forecasts for development of domiciliary services. Major capital spending is planned in the Scottish psychiatric hospitals (Scottish Working Group, 1984, 1985; Scottish Home and Health Department, 1985); this is contrary to the expressed Scottish Health Authorities Priorities for the Eighties Report ('SHAPE', Scottish Home and Health Department, 1980b), which suggested that the large psychiatric hospitals should be reduced in size and small units be provided in reasonable proximity to the population they serve.

Somewhat paradoxically, the lack of clarity of definition may be responsible for the term's durability and attractiveness. Walker (1982) comments:

'This lack of clarity is crucial in explaining the form that community care policies have taken, because it suggests different conceptions of *need* at different times and in relation to different groups.'

Arie (1972) called this vagueness 'semantic plasticity'. The definitions used in policy documents however, can be classified into three types of definition: administrative, sociological and moral.

The *administrative* definitions tend to detail the resources to be developed and often emphasise care provision by the statutory and professional organisations. For example:

> 'In this document the term "Community" covers a whole range of provision including hospitals, hostels, day hospitals, residential homes, day care and domiciliary support. The term community care embraces primary health care and all the above services whether provided by health authority or local authorities ...' (Department of Health and Social Security, 1977)

The *sociological* definitions tend to be all-embracing and emphasise the role of and the caring capacity of society. For example:

> '... to help people live an independent life in their own homes for as long as possible.' (Department of Health and Social Security, 1976)

The *moral* definitions tend to emphasise 'what is best' and focus on the role of lay carers and voluntary organisations:

> '... to maintain a person's link with family, friends and normal life and to offer the support that meets his or her particular needs. Most people who need long term care can and should be looked after in the community. This is what most of them want for themselves and what those responsible for their care believe to be best.' (Department of Health and Social Security, 1981a)

These definitions are analogous to discussions of care *in, for* and *by* the community, each of which is elaborated below.

Despite the apparent agreement, then, about the 'goal' of 'community care', closer examination reveals that different people may not share the same view about the meaning of the concept: 'community care' means different things at different times and in relation to different groups in need. 'Community care' in relation to specific client groups has been the subject of considerable attention but much less effort has been devoted to an overall analysis of the development of community care (Department of Health and Social Security, 1981b).

Notwithstanding the conflicting definitions, it is worth exploring the concept of 'community care' further. This examination begins by looking at what care is like *in* the community setting. Care *for* the community is then focused on, and, finally, what care *by* the community really means.

Care in the community

In the following paragraphs some of the literature on resource allocation within the health service generally is examined. Psychiatric care provision is then focused on, emphasising the situation in Scotland. This reveals that there is a need to develop services outside hospital provision.

Community care policy and practice compared

Community care appears to be political rhetoric, rather than practical reality. This is borne out by the figures on resource allocation and use within the health service generally, which illustrate that resource allocation is still hospital-bound rather than community orientated (Royal Commission on the National Health Service, 1979, Haywood and Alaszewski, 1980). The Social Services Committee Report (1985, p.xvi, para. 24) talks of the impending 'crisis in the community' as far as psychiatry is concerned: '90% of care is provided by psychiatric hospitals while 90% of patients are in the community.' This reflects a preoccupation with hospital care, to the relative neglect of those outside hospital.

Looking at resource allocation in relation to specialities within the health service, it is clear that resources continue to be channelled into the high-technology, curative services rather than into the care of the long-term chronic sick. This is despite the facts that around half of the hospital beds are occupied by long-stay patients – elderly, mentally-handicapped and the mentally ill – and that most people use and consult the community-based health facilities (Salvage, 1985). Townsend (1981) further illustrates that there are more than twice as many bed-fast and severely-disabled people living in their own homes as in all the institutions put together.

In Britain at large community care services have been adversely affected by recent cuts in public spending (Walker et al, 1979; Personal Social Services Council, 1979; Politics of Health Group, undated). Co-ordination between different services is quoted as being a vital component of community care (Department of Health and Social Security, 1971, 1974, 1976, 1981). As Walker (1982) has commented, collaboration is a poor substitute for lack of resources.

Lack of community resources

The deficiency and shortfalls of service provision, contrary to official guidelines, have been well documented in official and independent reports (see Townsend and Davison, 1982, as regards general health; Topliss and Gould, 1981, with regard to the disabled; Wertheimer, 1982, for the mentally handicapped; Hunt, 1978, for the elderly). As regards psychiatry, the Social Services Committee refers to 'the cart before the horse phenomenon' as being the hallmark of community care policies, where psychiatric hospital closures are pushed for without the provision of an alternative infrastructure of community services (Social Services Committee, 1985 p.xviii, para. 30). Brook and Cooper (1975) talk of the 'impending crisis' in psychiatry in which:

'Paradoxically, increased demands have arisen largely as a result of the trend towards community care for the mentally ill, which while reducing the numbers of mental hospital beds, has at the same time created a need for greatly expanded out-patient, day patient and domiciliary care. The burden on hospital psychiatry has become all the heavier because of the tardiness of local authorities in providing, and of central government in financing, residential and day care placements for patients with chronic disabilities.'

More recently, the Audit Commission (1986) has recommended radical changes in organising community care in order to avoid 'a continued waste of scarce resources and, worse still, care and support that is either lacking entirely, or inappropriate to the needs of some of the most disadvantaged members of society and the relatives who seek to care for them.'

Care of the mentally ill in Scotland: hospital orientation of service
Care of the mentally ill in Scotland is more hospital-orientated than that in other parts of the UK. This hospital orientation partly reflects Scotland's more guarded commitment to community care which is apparent in policy statements: Scotland unlike England is not pursuing a policy of hospital closure (Scottish Home and Health Department, 1985; Scottish Working Group, 1984, 1985). These documents provide evidence of the divergence of Scottish policy from that of the rest of Britain. The Department of Health for Scotland, 1962, recommended a running down of the psychiatric hospitals, whereas England and Wales' Hospital Plan of the same year envisaged eventual hospital closure.) Closure of mental hospitals has given impetus to the debate on community care elsewhere, e.g. the 'Italian experience' (Jones and Poletti, 1985) and the American policy of 'deinstitutionalisation' (Brown 1985b), in an attempt to focus attention on alternative forms of care and to learn from the experience of others.

Shortfall in Scottish psychiatric community services
Clarke (1982), The Mental Welfare Commission (1981, 1986), and Mental Health in Focus (Scottish Home and Health Department, 1985) have all discussed shortfalls in the provision of services in relation to the mentally ill in Scotland. The most recent Scottish policy document referring to care of the mentally ill points out that there are serious shortfalls in the present service provision for meeting current demand: 3700 day places are urgently needed and outpatient clinics and increased involvement with primary care teams are major recommendations. A major injection of funding and reorientation of resources is required to meet present day demands (Scottish Home and Health Department, 1985). The Scottish Health Service Planning Council produced a national programme of health

priorities for the eighties (The SHAPE Report, Scottish Home and Health Department, 1980b) which identified the mentally ill as a 'category A' priority target group. This report followed on from 'The Way Ahead' (Scottish Home and Health Department, 1976) but the SHAPE Report differed from the first document in that SHHD intended to monitor the progress of the implementation of SHAPE recommendations (Scottish Home and Health Department, 1985). Yet, according to a Scottish Working Group Report (1984), by 1984 only four of the 15 Scottish Health Boards had produced complete planning statements and the remainder were unavailable for public discussion. Three examples below demonstrate that there is a need for services to be developed in the community to improve the standards of care for the mentally ill in Scotland.

1. Demographic trends show that elderly people are more prone to becoming mentally ill than are younger adults. At present almost 17% of the population in Scotland is of pensionable age and 41% of old people living on their own are over 75. Twenty-five per cent of old people in Scotland have no children and 22% have no brothers or sisters. Only a very small proportion of old people is in hospital or residential care – 5%. Clearly these figures lend support to the notion of a more community-orientated psychiatric service where there is a varied and larger variety of resources and treatments available. In the next 10 years the proportion of the over-75s will have increased by 36%. These figures (Age Concern, 1984) also suggest that, in the future, statutory services and 24-hour care will be in greater demand.

2. A recent Scottish survey of 'new chronic inpatients' (psychiatric patients aged 18–64 who on the census date had been in hospital for more than one year but less than six years), in 14 Scottish hospitals, found that 38% of the patients did not need to be in hospital if alternative accommodation was available (McCreadie et al, 1983).

3. In a recent report, the Mental Welfare Commission (1986) suggested that there are a group of 'entrapped patients' who:

> 'are detained in hospitals simply because there is no alternative means of caring for them and in whose case no feature of their condition makes it necessary that they should continue to be in hospital.'

This issue has been identified as a matter of concern, is currently being investigated by the Commission and will be the subject of a future report.

The above summary on aspects of care *in* the community demonstrates that there is a lack of provision outside the hospital, i.e. in the community setting. This applies throughout the National Health Service but is especially true of Scottish psychiatry. As it exists, community care is inadequately provided for the mentally ill. Present community resources should be expanded to meet projected needs. Lack of shifts in this direction suggest that the health service is not serious about providing psychiatric care *in* the community. These points are emphasised in a recent publication by the Scottish Association for Mental Health, which reviews the community mental health services in Scotland (Drucker, 1987).

Care for the community

Care *for* the community reflects the broadest interpretations of the concept and refers to increasing the caring potential of 'the community' at large. The idea of increasing the caring potential of 'the community' has proved an attractive approach to politicians against a background of the health-care system which is suffering decline (Walker, 1982), and which has been criticised in recent years both for failing to promote egalitarianism and to improve the health and life experiences of deprived groups (Wilding and George, 1984), and for being inefficient and wasteful (Department of Health and Social Security, 1983). This interpretation of 'community care' underpins current political thinking, as shown by the Conservative Party Manifesto, quoted in Brenton (1985):

> 'In the community we must do more to help people to help themselves, and families to look after their own. We must also encourage the voluntary movement and self-help groups working in partnership with the statutory agencies.'

Brenton continues, and comments '. . . this [focus on helping people to help themselves] has served to focus attention on the government's enthusiastic subscription to the ethos of community care, giving this form of care a new moral and ideological justification for the 1980's.' Brenton further demonstrates that this view is common among politicans, regardless of party allegiance:

> 'The growing political interest in the potential of voluntary social services may be directly linked to the desire to make economies in the public sector. Any searching examination of successive policy statements in recent years finds abundant evidence for this link, but it does not explain the whole story. In the rediscovery by politicians of the virtues of the voluntary sector, one may also detect, besides a preoccupation with the expenditure consequences of recession, the adoption and strengthening of distinct ideological positions. Labour ministers, particularly those with responsibilities for social services, shifted towards accepting that the voluntary sector could and should play a valuable complementary role alongside the main-line statutory services, and here they became virtually indistinguishable from the left of the Conservative Party. It is probably fair to say that economies in social expenditure remained the uppermost consideration and that this ideological shift for Labour contained a large dose of pragmatism. Nevertheless, the party had moved in the direction of 'welfare pluralism' both practically and rhetorically by the time the Thatcher government came to power to pursue a rather more drastic reappraisal of the role of the state.'

This extract is quoted at length as it epitomises current political issues which, combined with the comments about the health service, are resulting in a 'reappraisal of the role of the state in social welfare' (Hadley and Hatch, 1982) and a move towards using voluntary agencies and others, instead of the state, to provide 'community care'. These issues are relevant to the work of community psychiatric nursing in that service organisers are being asked to evaluate the work for which they have managerial accountability (see p.33).

Walker (1982) reviews the adverse impact of state policies on the caring capacity of the community, and he comments that few measures have been introduced to support the caring activities of families. He argues that 'an increase in the caring capacity of the community requires action on employment, the relationship between sex and the labour market, housing, urban decay, incomes and public expenditure in order to promote a less hostile environment in which caring relationships can develop'. Walker advocates that future services should be based on the expressed need of carers and those being cared for, that these should be flexible and that this would require a collaboration on the part of health and social service professionals to allow central planning and local initiatives to be reconciled. Major questions remain about whether or not these proposals could be possible.

Three interpretations of 'community care' were noted by Sladden (1979):

'1. as care of social problems by social agencies.
2. as any care or treatment which does not involve hospital admission.
3. as a comprehensive system of preventative psychiatry.'

The latter formulation is based on Caplan's three-fold classification of preventative psychiatry (Caplan, 1964):

'which refers to the body of professional knowledge, both theoretical and practical which may be utilised to plan and carry out programs for the reduction of:

1. the incidence of mental disorders of all types in the community – primary prevention;
2. the duration of a significant number of those disorders which do occur – secondary prevention;
3. the impairment which may result from those disorders – tertiary prevention.'

The first two interpretations noted by Sladden (1979) reflect the established patterns of psychiatric treatment in Britain where social and other approaches to care (mainly medical) are split off and separated (Penfold and Walker, 1983). This is mirrored at the national level by the separate development of health and social services.

The final interpretation is relevant to this discussion about 'care for the community'. This takes quite a different approach to care – prevention is introduced into the picture and concern focuses on groups of people as well as individuals. Caplan's model, which embraces primary, secondary and tertiary prevention, implies that community care should be concerned as much with groups of populations as with individuals. Bellak (1964) has commented:

> 'The preventive ideology requires the acceptance of responsibilities extending beyond the normal range of clinical functions to quasi-political community action.'

It is debatable whether or not this approach to 'community care' can be taken by professionals and particularly by community psychiatric nurses. Current knowledge of causal factors in psychiatry is incomplete, for example, and it is, therefore, doubtful whether preventative approaches can be taken in psychiatry. Furthermore, professional training and practice are also generally focused on individuals (Hunter, 1978), not on groups, so it is unclear whether and how professionals and community psychiatric nurses are prepared for this role. There is in fact some evidence that taking a preventative approach in communities can have adverse effects: Cumming and Cumming (1957) found that the community tends not to be amenable to health education, and Sarbin and Mancuso (1970) have shown that the public's increased awareness of illness and health education leads to reduced tolerance and increased diagnosing.

This 'preventative' approach appears to be gaining influence in contemporary psychiatry in Britain, as evidenced by the attention given to social factors which are acknowledged as an influence on treatment and outcome (see Brown and Harris, 1978, and p.26 about how this affects the work of community psychiatric nursing). Combined with the increased availability of drugs, these developments have led to an increased realisation of the therapeutic and rehabilitative potential of the community setting itself.

Care by the community

Closer examination of the term 'community care' reveals that this is a value-laden concept (Wilson, 1982) because care *by* the community is considered desirable and, furthermore, preferable to institutional care. It is also assumed that this care outside the institution will be with a family. These assumptions are explored, then challenged.

The assumption of the desirability of care by *the community*
In general 'community' is linked with images of the good life – of what is desirable and thought to promote intimacy and stability. There is nostalgia for the romantic image of village life with its

healthy people and perfect forms of social control, where people pass on wisdom to successive generations, and mutual respect and support are the norm. This is set against the image of the metropolis and the industrial, uncaring city, where people mingle impersonally, where life is organised contractually and judicially rather than according to tradition, and where disorganisation and disintegration is the order of the day. The findings of Barton (1959) and Goffman (1961), and a catalogue of hospital enquiries (see Department of Health and Social Security, 1974; Martin, 1984), gave an impetus to discussions on the supremacy of community care over institutional care. The debate has tended to degenerate into a good/bad dichotomy, reflecting the enduring and emotive imagery described above. Proof of the power of this polarisation in favour of community care is illustrated by the preoccupation of policy documents with community care, geared to avoid 'institutionalisation', at the expense of discussing hospital care options.

The assumption of 'the family'

The current Prime Minister, Margaret Thatcher, has described the 'welfare state' as the 'nanny state', and has argued on economic grounds to cut expenditure on the health and social services. Under-pinning the economic arguments is the accusation that the welfare state is over-collectivised and has diminished the vital freedoms and choices of individuals. Contained within this ideology is an appeal to values deeply embedded in nineteenth-century traditions of liberal political economy with their heavy emphasis on individual achievement and effort as a measure of social deservingness. Moralistic Tory notions of the family as a primary source of authority and assistance combine with an accent on other forms of decentralised social responsibility radically to shift the locus of collective obligation away from the state and central government towards care (of dependents) by 'the family'.

Wilson (1982) points out that 'the family' has become imbued with the valued qualities associated with community life. This means that the family has accordingly become poised against the opposite notion of the institution, with its less attractive sequelae (see Barton, 1959). The integrity of the family has become one of the central assumptions of community care; the family is assumed to be responsible for care of dependents and it is assumed that the family is a cohesive and caring unit.

The assumptions behind community care are rarely stated in the literature, far less questioned. Exceptions to this statement are Hawks (1975) and Ashton (1978). Hawks suggests that the commitment to a policy of community care which favours decentralisation, delegation and participation could be the result of medicine's redefining areas of responsibility. It may also be related to the increased difficulties of staffing hospitals, as is also suggested by the comments of the Social Services Committee Report (1985).

The assumptions described above can be challenged as described below.

The myth of the desirability of community care
The work of Barton (1959) and Goffman (1961) emphasised the institutional roots of much disordered behaviour which was previously believed to be an inevitable part of the course of chronic psychiatric illness. These authors showed that institutional care can produce 'institutional neurosis', characterised by symptoms of apathy, lack of initiative and loss of interest. This loss of interest is particularly marked in relation to personal possessions and the present. There is also an apparent lack of interest in and an ability to plan for the future. Barton (1959) lists several factors which are associated with the development of institutional neurosis: loss of contact with the outside world; enforced idleness; unsuitable staff behaviour (particularly bossiness, brow-beating, brutality and teasing); bad ward atmosphere; loss of personal friends; drug effects; and the loss of prospects outside the institution.

Wing and Brown (1961) surveyed female schizophrenic patients in three psychiatric hospitals and found that poverty of the social environment (few personal possessions, pessimistic nurses and little contact with the outside world) was associated with most clinical disturbance. In a further account of the same study, Wing and Brown (1970) found that the most important single factor associated with clinical improvement was a reduction in the time spent doing nothing. The category which distinguished patients who improved was 'work and occupational therapy'. A desire to avoid 'institutionalisation' or the development of 'institutional neurosis' has been a major reason given for the (allegedly preferable) development of community care.

Milverton (1985), however, has argued that the factors associated with the production of institutionalisation can also be found in patients who are cared for in their own homes, and that patients can become institutionalised outside the hospital ward. Freeman and Simmons (1958) also described the family home which could resemble 'a one-person chronic' ward. This suggestion is founded on observation rather than systematic study.

Little systematic information is available about the routine of patients in the home setting. Brown et al (1966), in a survey of discharged hospital patients, found that many patients spent large amounts of time doing nothing. This could be considered similar to the 'enforced idleness' mentioned by Barton and, hence, taken to be evidence of the existence of 'institutional neurosis' outside the hospital.

Hawks (1975) believes that institutionalisation is not an issue in today's hospitals, and that facilities for rehabilitation and social training far surpass those available in the community. Evidence of lack of community facilities may provide some support for Hawk's opinion.

More information is needed about the development of secondary handicap outside the institution. There is no evidence that shows the effect of community psychiatric nursing contact (or, for that matter, other types of intervention) on the discharged patients' risk of developing 'institutional neurosis'. More information is needed on this. It cannot be categorically stated that secondary handicap will not develop in the home situation; current evidence, in the form of shortage of resources, could suggest that it might. Home care then is not necessarily 'better' than institutional care.

The myth of the cohesive and caring family

There is some evidence that the social security system is being eroded by deliberate government policy and inflation (Salvage, 1985). Families find it hard to survive, and hardship may lead to domestic violence, divorce, and children being taken into care. The rise in unemployment does little to foster family harmony, and the present government's policy of encouraging migration in search of jobs probably tends to undermine family cohesion. The increase in one-parent families, divorces and second marriages (and second families), combined with an increase in the number of women working (despite the recession; Gardiner, 1981), all affect the family's capacity to care. Contemporary families, as described, may not be the cohesive unit that one is led to believe.

The myth of the family unit

A family, by definition, is a group of people. In reality, 'caring' does not embrace the family 'as a group'. In practice, it is the female kin who overwhelmingly care for the dependents (Townsend, 1981; Equal Opportunities Commission, 1982a,b). This reflects the sexual division of labour in our society where women are predominantly associated with the private sphere of work – in the house – and men, the public sphere – outside the home (Miller, 1976). Elizabeth Wilson summarises this argument (Wilson, 1982):

'The community is an ideological portmanteau word for a reactionary, conservative ideology that oppresses women by silently confining them to the private sphere without so much as even mentioning them. Moreover, it attempts to confine them, or at least implicitly to define them, at the same time as economic policy and social change pushes them into the public sphere of paid work, and yet simultaneously removes the last state props that supported them in their work in the "community", that is in the family.'

Care *by* the community is, then, in a very real sense being undertaken by female kin (often called 'informal carers'); friends and voluntary groups also assume a significant role in the provision of care. An extensive debate on the definition and role of voluntary organisations is not appropriate here (see the Wolfenden Committee Report, 1978, and Brenton, 1985, for details); suffice it to say that there has been an upsurge of interest in the potential of voluntary agencies in the care of the mentally ill in recent years, and that voluntary agencies also do valued and varied work. A classification by function of voluntary groups suggests the following typology: a service-providing function; a mutual aid function; a pressure group function; a resource function; and a co-ordinating function.

It is a matter of urgency that the contribution of these non-governmental carers be acknowledged and particularly so with the curtailment of the care-giving capacity of contemporary women. Professional carers, at least, should be supporting the lay carers in this role. There is some evidence that moves are being made in this direction (see Scottish Action on Dementia Report, 1986a, b). Recent policy documents refer to 'partnerships' between the statutory and voluntary sectors (Department of Health and Social Security, 1977), and the emphasis on 'joint planning' approaches to care provision points to potential areas of joint action and combined effort (Scottish Home and Health Department, 1985). Involvement of these groups could result in a more consistent approach to supporting informal networks, provide a more comprehensive system of care and allow for joint initiatives.

It seems that 'community care' policies have been restricted in conception, limited in application and based on often unacceptable assumptions about the duty, willingness and ability of families (and women in particular) to care for dependents. This can no longer be considered a sound basis for providing community care.

Sladden (1979) further comments on 'community care':

> 'Unless these divergent interpretations of community care are recognised and until a common approach is evolved, it is inevitable that there will be uncertainty and confusion about the contributions of the community psychiatric nurse.'

In the following two sections the work of community psychiatric nursing is examined and the relevant literature on this speciality reviewed.

THE WORK OF COMMUNITY PSYCHIATRIC NURSING

This thesis is concerned with examination of the 'process' of community psychiatric nursing, what the nurses are doing. This also involves the notion of 'functioning', in a sociological sense, which may be used to describe the activity of an object or entity which fulfils some purpose. The term also has a second application, where it means the objective consequences of some social action or phenomenon. The consequences of such action may be intended and recognised by those involved, in which case the function is 'manifest'; alternatively the consequences may be unintended and unrecognised, in which case the function is 'latent'. In this sense, use of the term 'functioning' is also appropriate for the present study which looks at the consequences of the work of the community psychiatric nurses.

In the next section, brief comment is made, first, about the historical development and, second, about the lack of a clear definition of community psychiatric nursing. The work of community psychiatric nursing is then detailed in order to present the theoretical framework surrounding the practice of community psychiatric nurses and in order to set the context for examination of the work of community psychiatric nursing.

Definitions of community psychiatric nursing

The historical development of community psychiatric nursing is reviewed by Baker (1968), Sladden (1979) and White and Mangan (1981). The development of community psychiatric nursing is explored and discussed further below. Hunter, in 1974, commented:

'Papers or comments in nursing journals on community psychiatric nursing have increased considerably even though much of what has been written is of a general nature, rather than descriptive of what the nurses or services are actually doing.'

This state of affairs has changed since the mid 1970s, and there has been an increase in the number of papers describing what community psychiatric nursing and services are actually doing (e.g. Roberts, 1976; Donnelly, 1977a; Ryce, 1978; Leopoldt, 1979a, b; Coverdale, 1980; Sharpe, 1980; Tough et al, 1980; Brough, 1982). These and other papers demonstrate that use of the term 'community psychiatric nurse' cannot be guaranteed to mean the same thing to different people. Some community psychiatric nurses work full time in the community (Leopoldt, 1974), whereas others assert that the job is so demanding that it can only be done part time (Warren, 1971; Maisey, 1975).

The work of community psychiatric nursing
In an attempt to detail the work of community psychiatric nursing, task-centred definitions have arisen. These demonstrate that there are differing opinions of what a community psychiatric nurse

should do: giving injections is considered a vital component of the work of the community psychiatric nurse by Nickerson (1972) and Warren (1971), and considered an 'informed contribution' by Leopoldt (1974); this activity is rejected as inappropriate by other authors (Stobie and Hopkins, 1972a, 1972b). Talking of Modecate clinics, Stobie and Hopkins comment that this therapy is most effectively carried out by the general practitioner with the help of a public health nurse.

It is possible that domiciliary visiting could be used as a defining characteristic of community psychiatric nursing, although it is acknowledged, as Pullen (1980) and Altschul (1972a, 1973) have noted, that other professionals apart from community psychiatric nurses are involved in domiciliary work with psychiatric patients. Some authors consider that domiciliary visiting is coterminous with community psychiatric nursing (Henderson et al, 1973), yet people called community psychiatric nurses work from various bases: (Elliot-Cannon, 1981) from a hospital base; (White, 1983) from a health-centre base; (Williamson et al, 1981) with district general hospital attachment; and all these CPNs may not necessarily be involved in home visiting (Kirkpatrick, 1967; MacDonald, 1972; Shires, 1977).

Conflicting statements can be found about community psychiatric nursing activities by authors from the psychiatric nursing field (Sencicle, 1981; Sharpe, 1982) and by other professionals (Baker, 1968; Henderson et al, 1973; Ritson, 1977; Hunter, 1980; Pullen, 1980; Tough et al, 1980; McKechnie et al, 1981). It may be that different services have different priorities about the value of certain activities. It is unclear whether community psychiatric nurses within any one service hold similar values about activities or whether they have a common rationale for their work. This issue is explored in the present study.

The practice of community psychiatric nursing

The majority of community psychiatric nurses are not specifically trained for work in the community setting (see p.57) and, accordingly, use models and theories learned during basic psychiatric nurse training. What follows is a brief review of the most common models and theories employed by psychiatric nurses and hence available for community psychiatric nurses' use.

The nursing process
Up until the 1960s, professional nursing practice seemed to be based on instinct and empathy. The publication of Yura and Walsh's book (1967) marked a turning point in nursing practice in that it introduced the 'nursing process' as a tool for clinical nurses; it is from this date that the practice of nursing has become more systematic. The

'nursing process' simply distinguished four clear stages in the provision of nursing care, namely, assessment, planning, goal-setting (and identification of nursing intervention or actions) and, finally, evaluation. This approach has been criticised in that 'it exhorts nurses to assess, but tells them little about what to assess. It encourages planning but says little about how to plan. It asks nurses to intervene, but fails to say in what ways. It advocates evaluation, but does not specify when or how' (Aggleton and Chalmers, 1986). Nevertheless, this approach to care remains the main prescriptive model used by most nurses.

Models of care in psychiatric nursing

A 'model' is described by Riehl and Roy (1980) as:

> 'a systematically constructed, scientifically based and logically related set of concepts which identify the essential components of nursing practice together with the theoretical basis of these concepts and values required for their use by the practitioner.'

Models (also called conceptual models) of nursing have a number of components on which they are likely to make some comment: the nature of people; the causes of problems likely to require nursing intervention; the nature of the assessment process; the nature of the planning and goal-setting process; the focus of intervention during the implementation of the care plan; the nature of the process of evaluating the quality and effects of the care given; and the role of the nurse. There are many models available to nurses, which can help in the provision of nursing care. For a summary of a range of nursing models see Aggleton and Chalmers (1986). The following pages briefly review those which are most commonly used by psychiatric nurses.

Burgess (1985) describes four major models which are widely used in psychiatric nursing: biological or medical, social, psychological, and behavioural. When a patient is being treated, the kind of assessment obtained, the meaning assigned to certain historical facts and the treatment methods used depend on which model is chosen.

The medical model The medical model forms the basis of most training (nursing and medical) in psychiatry (Drucker, 1987) and results in the efforts of clinicians being directed towards the identification of physiological malfunctions and chemical imbalances. A person's social behaviour and psychological process are thought to originate from physiological and biological activities. This reductionist view has been criticised as it encourages an understanding of people as 'passive hosts of disease' (Reynolds, 1985) and provides an illness-orientated approach to care. Assessment is designed to determine what is medically wrong with the person and focuses on signs and symptoms which are usually obtained by taking a medical history and physically examining the patient. This process of assessment leads to a 'diagnosis' being made of a medical 'condition' and results in a plan of care in which treatment is prescribed (usually by doctors) to rectify the malfunction. Nurses in the medical model can find themselves as accessories to medicine and taking on a handmaiden role to doctors. Reed and Lomas (1984) talked about 'closed referral systems' in community services (that is, community psychiatric nursing services which only receive referrals from consultant psychiatrists), and said that these perpetuate a line of accountability to the doctors who in fact prescribe nursing intervention.

The social model   The social model of treatment has historical roots in the 'moral treatment' of the nineteenth century, where the emphasis was on the development of 'friendly association, discussion of his [the patient's] difficulties and the daily pursuit of purposeful activity' (Rees, 1957). The social view of psychiatric illness focuses on the way the individual functions in the social system. Treatment consists of reorganising the patient's relationship to the social system or reorganising the social system (for example, if an individual's behaviour is irrational he can be helped to stop acting in this way or the family can be helped better to tolerate the behaviour). Nursing intervention may include the creation of a therapeutic milieu, aiding the patient to improve his or her social skills and competencies, focusing on patient's difficulties in a problem-orientated way or establishing relationships with individuals to help them to express their feelings and cope with their emotions. Using this model, the patient and nurse jointly negotiate the goals of nursing intervention.

The psychological model   The psychological model stems from the work of Sigmund Freud, and has as its basis the belief that psychological disturbances are understandable and result from childhood experiences and distortions of reality which lead to impaired personality development and inappropriate behaviour. Nursing intervention includes group and individual psychotherapy in order to help the patient to gain a better understanding of himself. The model includes the nurse helping the patient to verbalise feelings instead of acting immediately; the nurse encourages patients to talk, listens to them and supports them through emotional experiences and change. This is well described in the following passage from Burgess (1981):

> 'Initially the nurse should start by just listening and trying to understand the human process within the person, instead of trying to concentrate on specific interviewing techniques contained in some textbooks ... The patient must know that the nurse is aware of his goals, his strivings and his wishes and that the nurse is working hard with him in order to accomplish these goals.'

This extract shows how the nurses use interpersonal theories (see below).

The behavioural model The behavioural model is the fourth model used by psychiatric nurses and rests on the conceptualisation of Pavlov's conditioned learning theory (for an elaboration of this and its use by psychiatric nurses, see Barker and Fraser, 1985). Using this model, abnormal behaviour is assumed to have been learned and is maintained because it has positive benefits or avoids negative consequences. Nursing activity is aimed at altering the overt (maladaptive) behaviour and teaching patients other, more appropriate, forms of behaviour.

The psychiatric nurse implicitly uses one or a combination of conceptual models to assess and plan patient care by the process referred to as 'clinical judgment'. The nurse may also be influenced by training, temperament, or her clinical bias (or that of the therapeutic setting) to see patients predominantly from one conceptual point of view. The decision to use one model often diminishes the possibility of using another model simultaneously. Psychiatric nurses have been described as taking an 'eclectic approach' to patients, where information derived from all models of care is used. The process of 'clinical judgment' results in planned care which is referred to as 'therapy'.

Theories in psychiatric nursing
Additionally, psychiatric nurses may use certain theories to facilitate practice (some of the theories on which the models have been based have already been mentioned). Theories have been defined by Chinn and Jacobs (1983) as:

'a set of concepts, definitions and propositions that project a systematic view of phenomena by designating specific interrelationships among concepts for purposes of describing, explaining, predicting and/or controlling phenomena.'

They are similar to models in that they are built up from ideas and concepts, but they are distinctive because they have an ability to explain and predict *specific* phenomena (Fawcett, 1984). There are few theories which have been developed from nursing knowledge; most theories used in nursing are borrowed from the other sciences. Two examples of theories used in psychiatry are particularly relevant to the work of community psychiatric nurses; these theories are interpersonal relationship theory (Rogers, 1957) and crisis intervention theory (Caplan, 1964).

Interpersonal relationship theory 'Building relationships' is a generally accepted premise on which psychiatric nursing is based (Altschul, 1972a; Cormack, 1976; Reynolds, 1985). Hildegard Peplau's work, defining the importance of interpersonal relations (Peplau, 1952), was a milestone in the development of a theoretical base for psychiatric nursing. Peplau proposed a descriptive conceptual framework which drew heavily on Sullivan's interpersonal theory and, to a lesser extent, on learning theory (Sullivan, 1953). This framework allows the nurse to help the patient to examine situational factors, with the focus on improving interpersonal competencies that have been lost or never learned.

The relationship between nurse and patient has been described as a 'caring relationship'. This is explored in numerous texts (for example, Downie and Telfer, 1980) and can only be given a brief mention here. The word 'relationship' is used in two ways: to stand for the situation, occasion or bond which links two or more people (e.g. marriage, business association or an emergency), or to stand for the attitude which people so linked have for each other (e.g. fear, pride, respect, love).

The bond which constitutes the nurse/patient 'relationship' consists of formal rules, both legal and administrative. For example, in psychiatry, nurses can retain a patient in hospital care if the patient - is a risk to himself or to others. There are other more vague sets of rules often referred to as the 'ethics' of the profession (for further details see Thompson et al, 1983). In nursing, these are enumerated in a nurses' Code of Professional Conduct (United Kingdom Central Council, 1984).

Additionally, certain kinds of attitudes are considered to accompany the development of a 'caring relationship'. The caring worker, for instance, should be *impartial* and as *objective* as possible in relation to the distribution of benefits in accordance with needs, and should be *non-judgmental* (Timms and Watson, 1978). Paradoxically, the nurse is discouraged from adopting a totally detached stance, but rather is encouraged to react to patients and help them to gain insight into their behaviour, and to hold an attitude of *compassion* (see Downie et al, 1974).

Psychiatric nurses are, in fact, explicitly taught that successful therapy is dependent upon the possession by the nurse of three facilitating conditions: warmth, empathy and genuineness (Rogers, 1957). This author suggested that aspects of personality and attitudes are crucial determinants of successful therapeutic outcome; he identified three essential attitudes which he suggested were critical factors in the therapeutic relationship: genuineness of human regard, a warm positive acceptance or non-judgmental approach to the patient, and a caring and empathic understanding of the patient. Clare and Thompson (1981) went one step further and stated that theoretical experience and knowledge are less relevant in influencing successful outcome than are personality factors. These attributes alone, regardless of model and therapy use, are considered vital components of the caring relationship. This is demonstrated clearly by the comments below:

> 'The quality of caring, as a genuine human concern, is important in the therapeutic alliance made with the patient. The patient must be made aware of the nurse's caring and must be convinced of the sincerity in order that definite progress may be made . . . Interest and caring about an individual are not technical skills; they are the basic arts of psychic healing.
>
> 'Nurses do not need to tell the patient they care. They show concern for the patient by listening and by trying to understand the anguish or loneliness in the patient's heart. When nurses are comfortable enough to enable them not to worry about interview technique, posture, facial expression, and speech, the natural concerns for people will begin to show. It is then that the patient will know that the nurse cares.'(Burgess, 1981)

The care shown by a nurse for a patient has been described as 'friend-like' behaviour (Downie and Telfer, 1980). The authors state, 'The value of befriending must not be underestimated. For the lonely and helpless, befriending can be a lifeline'. The nurse, in fact, has a difficult task of being both objective and impartial, yet caring and compassionate.

The difficulties surrounding the development of 'nurse/patient relationships' are discussed at length by Schwartz and Shockley (1956) and by Brown and Pedder (1979). The latter authors distinguish three elements in the development of the nurse/patient relationship: the working alliance, transference and counter-transference. The former component resembles that discussed above; the latter two concepts refer to the emotional feelings of both nurse and patient, arising out of the caring relationship, which affect therapy and can lead to patient dependency. Nurses are warned against getting too involved, showing too much compassion and concern for patients, although helping patients (often in distress) and responding to them as individuals means, by necessity, that nurses must 'get involved' (Schwartz and Shockley, 1956).

Crisis intervention theory Caplan's three-fold classification of mental illness (Caplan 1964) is a theory which advocates that psychiatric workers be involved in preventative work aimed firstly at reducing the incidence of mental illness (primary prevention), secondly, at reducing the duration of disorders (secondary prevention) and, thirdly, at reducing the impairment that results from mental illness (tertiary prevention). This theory has implications for the work of community psychiatric nurses and legitimises work with a variety of individuals in varied settings.

Caplan's theory has given rise to questions about whether or not 'primary prevention' is feasible in psychiatry. Some authors are sceptical of this (see p.18), while others assert that primary prevention of mental illness is possible by aiming to minimise parents' anxiety, before transmission to the next generation (Denham, 1972). Pilkington (1973) claims that it is not possible to deal with chronic illness without becoming involved in the value systems of a society and devising means to influence them.

The Short Report (Social Services Committee, 1985), however, suggests that the function of psychiatric services in primary prevention is a chimera and implies that community psychiatric nurses should be headed away from such ambitions.

With regard to secondary and tertiary prevention, the literature indicates that it is not known whether early contact specifically with community psychiatric nurses is preferable to later contact, although, in relation to psychiatric treatment generally, there is substantial evidence in favour of early intervention (see Orford, 1987; Ratna, undated). The CPNA Survey (Community Psychiatric Nurses Association, 1985b) says that the majority of community psychiatric nurses are hospital-based (although there is considerable regional variation in this pattern). This could suggest that most community psychiatric nursing services are focusing on later, rather than early, treatment of mental distress (Goldberg and Huxley, 1980), and it could be argued that they are dealing with secondary and tertiary preventative activities.

From his initial theory, Caplan elaborated a 'crisis intervention approach' to care, which advocated that the optimum time to treat individuals in emotional distress (in order to effect change) was when they were in 'crisis'. Using crisis intervention theory allows nurses to legitimise work during crisis only (Langsley et al, 1969). This latter approach to care has resulted in nurses establishing drop-in centres and crisis counselling services (Oldfield, 1983) and using brief, time-limited approaches to treatment of patients (Fisch et al, 1982). Short spells in hospital have been used in the same way, in order to resolve crisis (Kennedy and Hird, 1980). This approach has been used in all three phases of preventative work.

Focusing on primary prevention and crisis work brings us to the concept of 'health education'. The community psychiatric nurse's work in relation to health education is a topic of concern in contemporary literature.

Nurses have taught people about health since the establishment of the profession. In the early days, the teaching reflected the general concern about sanitation and living conditions: Florence Nightingale (1859) emphasised that ill-health was the result of lack of whitewashing and ventilation, as well as of careless diet and dress. Cohen (1981) and Redman (1980), more recently, have carried out reviews of how the nurse's educational role is perceived. These indicate that nurses accept that they have a health education role but that there is confusion over the extent and nature of the activity required and uncertainty about how the nurse's role complements that of the doctor. Hunter (1978) found that community psychiatric nurses created opportunities for education of both families and patients.

It seems that, on an individual basis, the nurse can use the nurse/patient relationship for health education. The nurse can identify gaps in the patient's knowledge, and gear information-giving to the social class, education and experiences of the individual patient. The Community Psychiatric Nurses Association (1985d) asserts that the community psychiatric nurse has an important part to play in health education, although its assertions are not backed by research evidence.

Health education can take place in all three phases of preventative work referred to by Caplan (1964).

Before ending this section, it is worth commenting on the skills of psychiatric nurses.

The skills of the psychiatric nurse

Sladden (1979) and Cormack (1976), among others, have reviewed the literature on the role of the psychiatric nurse. The skills of the psychiatric nurse have been difficult to identify in the practical situation. Goddard (1955) used a job analysis method to look at the work of the psychiatric nurse and recommended (Goddard, 1958) that continuous observation studies of psychiatric nurses' duties needed to be made against the background environment and conditions in which the job was performed. Observation was a feature of later studies on psychiatric nursing, e.g. Oppenheim and Eeman (1955), John (1961), Cormack (1976) and Altschul (1972b); these all failed to investigate the subjective meaning which nurses ascribe to their own practice. Towell (1975) rectified this omission by taking a sociological approach to the work of psychiatric nurses (in three different hospital wards); the emphasis of the enquiry was on common roles and experiences of, rather than on the individual differences between, the nurses. Studies which have succeeded in identifying some of the skills and activities of the psychiatric nurse are reviewed below.

John (1961) used the medical model (which reflected her general nurse training) to examine the work of psychiatric nurses in four Scottish hospitals. She found that psychiatric nurses did not attend to the physical needs of their patients. Her study can be criticised on the grounds that she failed to make explicit the rationale for selecting her data.

McIlwaine (1980), who focused on the care of neurotic patients, found, by comparing psychiatric nurses and patient's perception of activities, that nurses were perceived as providers of pills, meals, support and reassurance. The personal qualities of the nurse were valued, as was the availability of the nurse to provide comfort in times of stress. McIlwaine's work emphasised the importance of the nurses' attitude in caring and showed that psychiatric nurses viewed neurotic patients negatively.

Identification of skills and activities that are particularly therapeutic is especially difficult. Cormack (1983) advanced knowledge in this direction by observing the behaviour of 14 charge nurses and classifying their behaviour into 23 codes. He also developed a questionnaire designed to measure patients' perceptions of psychiatric nurses. This was developed from comments using critical incident technique, and derived from a group of psychiatric nurses whom he neither described nor defined. Cormack believed that these perceptions were in themselves a measure of the nurses' therapeutic value. What he in fact derived was a measure of the process of psychiatric nursing in hospital, rather than a measurement of patient outcome or patient perception of therapeutic value. He focused on the interpersonal skills of psychiatric nurses and analysed his finding within a framework of goals. He considered that interpersonal skills of psychiatric nurses were used to reach three major types of goal:

1. direct goals (formal, where specific and predetermined goals were usually known to both the patient and the nurse);
2. direct goals (informal, where vague goals were used which were not necessarily known to the patient and nurse);
3. indirect goals (where the nurse acted as a facilitator for other professionals and allowed them to reach their goals).

Cormack found that psychiatric nurses minimally used interpersonal skills in the formal and structured sense. Virtually all examples of the effective use of interpersonal skills were of the direct goal (informal) and indirect goal types. Cormack's work stands out, in that it is the first piece of research which focused on and identified the interpersonal skills used by psychiatric nurses.

As we saw earlier, the personality and attitude of the nurse, rather than skills acquisition, may be a crucial factor in the development of the nurse/patient relationship. Shanley regarded the approach of Rogers (1957) as a 'skill' and examined the therapeutic interactions of psychiatric nurses to explore the nurses' possession of empathy, unconditional regard and genuineness. He also examined how charge nurses evaluated student nurses, and developed an inventory to look at the relationships that patients developed with nurses. Like Cormack's study (1976), this study focused on the patient's perception of 'process'. Shanley (1984) found that 90% of nurses had relationships that offered facilitative conditions for therapeutic change in patients (by implication, one in ten nurses did or do not). The nurses offered higher levels of the facilitative conditions to women than men and to depressed rather than schizophrenic patients. Unconditionality of regard received the lowest score, and it is unclear how this contributed to the relationship between nurse and patient.

Despite confusion about what skills psychiatric nurses possess, there is a general consensus that psychiatric nurses, by virtue of their training, provide a beneficial contribution to the care of the mentally ill. The CPNA Survey (Community Psychiatric Nurses Association, 1985b), showed that the majority of community psychiatric nurses were not specifically trained for community work, so it is reasonable to assume that community psychiatric nurses use the skills, models and theories acquired from their initial hospital-based training. This section has summarised those approaches used by psychiatric nurses who work in the community setting. It is unclear whether nurses develop or acquire new skills from the experience of community work. An examination of the work of community psychiatric nursing from the viewpoint of the nurses may help to clarify knowledge in this area.

EVALUATION OF COMMUNITY PSYCHIATRIC NURSING

The literature on community psychiatric nursing

Community psychiatric nursing literature is either descriptive or evaluative in nature.

Descriptive literature
Much of the writing on community psychiatric nursing is anecdotal and descriptive. Although lacking in objectivity, these reports provide a valuable measure of the scale of development of community psychiatric nursing and the form which this is taking. They also demonstrate the enthusiasm of individual practitioners and services to share experiences in an attempt to build up a body of knowledge about community psychiatric nursing. The concern to document the work of individual community psychiatric nurses does not seem to have been matched by a broad examination of resources being applied to community psychiatric nursing activity, and it is not clear how far existing knowledge of community psychiatric nursing is being utilised by service managers in evaluating the effectiveness of such services.

Recent papers repeatedly bemoan the excess of descriptive work and comment on the necessity to evaluate community psychiatric nursing services (Leopoldt and Hurn, 1973; Griffith and Mangen, 1980; Mangen and Griffith, 1982a,b; Paykel et al, 1982; Brooker,

1984b). As Leopoldt (1975) commented, 'Amount of work is neither a measure of its effectiveness nor its necessity'. Due to the excess of descriptive work examining community psychiatric nursing, it was determined that the emphasis of the present study be on evaluation.

Evaluative literature

The literature evaluating the work of community psychiatric nursing is reviewed below. Suchman (1967) proposed a distinction between evaluation and evaluation research. He defines 'evaluation' as, 'the general process of judging the worthwhileness of some activity regardless of the method employed', and 'evaluation research' as, 'the specific use of the scientific method for the purpose of making an evaluation'. This distinction separates 'evaluation', as a goal, from 'evaluation research', as a particular means of attaining that goal. As Luker (1982) comments:

> 'Evaluation when used in a general way is said to refer to the everyday occurrence of making judgements of worth. Although this interpretation implies some form of logical or rational thought it does not presuppose any systematic procedures of presenting objective evidence to support the judgement; evaluation when used in this way, refers only to the process of assessment or appraisal of worth.'

Use of the word 'research' implies systematic academic study which should be distinguished from non-systematic, journalistic description. Suchman's distinction facilitates examination of the literature on community psychiatric nursing. Many authors have evaluated the work of the community psychiatric nurse in Suchman's terms, but few have carried out evaluation research.

The literature and evaluation

Warren (1971) seems to have been one of the first authors who attempted to evaluate the work of the community psychiatric nurse. He took a 1 in 10 sample of patients receiving intramuscular injections from community psychiatric nurses' caseloads; he examined these patients' histories and found that those on medication had had fewer admissions since starting the injections. He assumed that the 'medication-giving' caused this reduced pattern of admission, and he then proceeded to calculate financial savings based on the hypothetical costs of admissions if the previous pattern had continued unabated. Warren concluded that the community psychiatric nursing service was cheaper. This study could not be considered a rigorous cost-benefit analysis as Warren compares marginal costs of community psychiatric nursing care with average costs of inpatient stay.

Jeevendrampillai (1982) also discussed costs of community psychiatric nursing and claimed that community psychiatric nursing was cheap. The author calculated the figure of £2.50 per hour as the cost of domiciliary care; it is not known how this figure was derived, and there are other costs of home care, such as support service and emotional costs, which are considered by Warren (1971).

Shaw (1977), a general practitioner, attempted to judge the worth of community psychiatric nursing by looking at the patients he had referred to the community psychiatric nurse over a six-month period, and presented a description of these patients by age, diagnosis and sex. He compared their management with the hypothetical management of patients in the absence of community psychiatric nursing, and concluded that the benefit to patients of community psychiatric nursing contact (compared with GP contact) were fewer prescriptions for psychotropic drugs and quicker psychiatric assessment (by community psychiatric nurses, rather than waiting for consultant or outpatient appointments). He concluded that the community psychiatric nursing care was better and cheaper.

Leopoldt et al (1974) described the experimental attachment of psychiatric nurses in health centres in Oxford and examined referral patterns and diagnostic groups. Harker et al (1976) reported on the same scheme and said that community psychiatric nurse attachments enhance patient care and reduce stigma. These studies, and those of Llewellyn (1974), Maisey (1975), Corrigan and Soni (1977), Sharpe (1980) and Brough (1982), all provide examples of studies which assert the worth of community psychiatric nursing by retrospectively examining referral patterns and admission rates, diagnosis and disposal of patients on community psychiatric nurses' caseloads. The authors tend to make assertions about the efficacy of community psychiatric nursing which are not entirely justified from the data, and alternative interpretations are possible. Llewellyn (1974), for example, regarded the fact of a developing service as evidence of a 'need' for community psychiatric nursing; the 'development' however, could be the result of other pressures and be unrelated to 'need'. Brough (1982) commented:

> 'These charts, apart from monitoring value, give a clear account of the services provided by community psychiatric nurses. It is not possible to say that it represents a need fulfilled as the nurses were working to full capacity and could not have met a higher demand.'

The charts do not, in fact, monitor value, although they give a vivid statistical analysis of changes in community psychiatric nursing provision over a specified time; there is also no evidence given to suggest that service development is related to specific needs. Corrigan and Soni (1977), Warren (1971) and Pullen (1980) all considered decrease in rates of hospital admission as an indication of 'successful' community psychiatric nursing intervention. Decrease in admissions could, of course, be caused by many factors – differing admission policies or varying criteria for admissions, for example – and not just by the work of the community psychiatric nurse. Pullen (1980) asserts that the problem-solving approach and 'family involvement' of domiciliary visits is 'useful' in one third of visits; no further elaboration of this is given (for what is it useful – providing background information, helping making treatment plans or avoiding the decision to admit?).

Another criticism that can be levelled at many 'evaluations' of community psychiatric nursing services is that reporters are often positively biased in favour of their own services. Pharaony and Mills (1976), for instance, questioned other disciplines about 'the need' for community psychiatric nurses. The author asked, 'Do you think there is a need for community psychiatric nurses, and if there was a service, would you refer?' For 'what' the community psychiatric nurses were needed was not detailed. The questions were biased towards gaining favourable answers about community psychiatric nursing. Balfour-Sclare (1971), similarly, lists seven prerequisites of the success of a community health project. The criteria are stated as a 'matter of fact', although they are the author's idea of success and are not necessarily valid as measures of success for all community psychiatric nursing services.

Diers (1979) has stated that 'without study the answer will be just guesswork'. Many of the studies discussed as 'evaluation' would be considered by Diers to be guesswork. The few studies which have used systematic approaches to acquire objective information are reviewed below. These would be included under Suchman's category of 'evaluation research'.

The literature and evaluation research

The framework of evaluation offered by Donabedian (1966), of 'structure–process–outcome', offers a skeleton around which community psychiatric nursing evaluation research can be discussed. The 'evaluation research' which focuses on each of these three areas in community psychiatric nursing is presented below.

Structure

Parnell (1974, 1978) conducted the first survey of community psychitric nursing which showed that service development in England and Wales lacked uniformity and that community psychiatric nurses worked from various bases and in varying capacities. Further surveys have illustrated that this picture remains valid today (Community Psychiatric Nurses Association 1981, 1985b). Although these surveys provide limited information on Scotland's community psychiatric nursing teams, they have yielded a 'snap-shot' of what community psychiatric nursing is doing at any one time. They have enabled identification of trends and issues of relevance to community psychiatric nursing and the wider field of psychiatry.

Skidmore and Friend (1984a–f) carried out interviews on 120 community psychiatric nurses from 12 community psychiatric nursing services in England. Their aim was to gain information on community psychiatric nursing in relation to specialism, education, enrolled nurses and community psychiatric nursing bases. They found that teams were shaped by the most dominant person in each and that community psychiatric nurses preferred a dual base. They reported that nurses preferred 'specialism' but questioned the benefit of this approach for the patients. They also found that community psychiatric nurses considered that they lacked skills, and concluded that education was necessary to improve this deficit. The absence of information about the methods of data collection, the interview schedule or the data analysis make appraisal of this study difficult.

Process

Process studies have generated detailed qualitative and quantitative information on community psychiatric nursing in specific occupational settings.

Altschul (1972a, 1973) conducted the first systematic study which examined what the community psychiatric nurse was actually doing. She studied the records available at Dingleton Hospital, conducted observation of domiciliary visits, and asked the professionals involved in these to complete a check-list of activities detailing aspects of this domiciliary care. The aim of the study was to investigate the multidisciplinary approach to the treatment of patients at home.

Altschul's study suggested that professionals' work overlaps in the home situation (as judged by the professionals concerned). She found that the community psychiatric nurse was responsible for the continuity of patient care and that it was community psychiatric nurses who arranged visits and completed the records. She found that only one in three teams provided information on support people present at interviews, and that a high proportion of visits were made to patients who lived alone. The community psychiatric nurses tended to ask questions about interpersonal relationships. The check-list results suggested that activities were not role-specific. Altschul also attempted to obtain detailed reports by nursing staff to try to identify the activities and the thinking behind them; this was abandoned because of the nurses' difficulty in talking in detail about their thoughts, feelings, perceptions and actions. Altschul's exemplary efforts to undertake an in-depth study of one psychiatric service suggested that it was unclear what skills community psychiatric nurses specifically offer in the domiciliary setting. This finding has since been corroborated in other studies.

Barker (1977) examines what the community psychiatric nurse is doing. Using diary analysis, Barker identified three areas of patient dependency and proposed a model on which community psychiatric nurses' work was based. The author also piloted a questionnaire to be used as an assessment tool following domiciliary visits. This appears to be one of the first studies introducing systematic assessment into community psychiatric nursing work.

Sladden (1977, 1979) described the activities of a group of hospital-based community psychiatric nurses, principally using interview technique and self-recording procedures. This study took a holistic approach to community psychiatric nursing and studied nurse – patient contacts in depth. Community psychiatric nursing practice was analysed: the data on domiciliary contacts were obtained from the nurses, and neither patients nor carers were asked for their opinions, only the referrers' and GPs' views of the service being obtained. Activities of the community psychiatric nurses fell into three distinct categories: medical treatment; psychological adjust-ment and social relationships; and socioeconomic problems and resources. Sladden suggested that domiciliary and outpatient clinic care were differentiated on two counts, first, by the use of different - frames of reference (outpatient work was related to a medical frame of reference and home care to a sociopsychological one), and second, by the fact that outpatient care was characterised by impersonal as opposed to individual type of care.

Harrison (1984) focused on community psychiatric nursing care of the elderly mentally infirm. He stated at the beginning of the questionnaire that he used in the study: 'We want to ask relatives about relatives' problems, patients about their problems and not conjectures on each other's behalf'. This laudable aim does not seem to have been achieved. The researcher developed a questionnaire which examined the community psychiatric nurses' views of pro-blems found in the patients. He found that all the patients had at least 10 problems, and some as many as 50. It is unclear from his research whether community psychiatric nursing involvement relieved these problems, or whether the community psychiatric nurse was unwilling or unable to take action to resolve the problems. It may be that some of the problems were not perceived as such by patients and relatives, and, therefore, no action by the community psychiatric nurse would be indicated (see Blaxter, 1976). Harrison's study provides valuable information on the social situation of the patients in the study: 32 out of the 69 had no caring relative living nearby, and 41 had less than one hour's daily contact with anyone at all. (For six patients, the community psychiatric nurse was the only visitor.)

McKendrick's work (1980,1981a,b; see p.61), surveyed the quan-titative measures used by services to measure performance. He found little consensus (between services) as to which aspects of care were recorded.

Statistical descriptions of community psychiatric nursing services can be considered here as they are attempts at quantifying the work of the community psychiatric nurse and at providing information on the 'process' of community psychiatric nursing. James (1961) refers to 'process' as, 'the number of times a bird flaps its wings without determination of how far he has flown'. This graphic description warns of the shortcoming of studying 'process' without consideration of 'outcome'. Outcome studies will now be discussed; in community psychiatric nursing they are notable by their scarcity

Outcomes

Hunter (1978), in a large scale five-year study of community psychiatric nursing care of schizophrenic patients, conducted the first outcome study of community psychiatric nurses. Mangen and Griffith (1982a) commented that:

> 'Hunter (1978) found that, retrospectively, community psychiatric nursing care was inferior to normal follow up, though one would have to be cautious in interpreting his data as there is a very real possibility that the patient samples were not adequately matched.'

This criticism is not entirely justified. Hunter compared two groups of patients, retrospectively matched by similarity of hospital background: one group received care from community psychiatric nurses, the other did not. He found that the patient cared for by community psychiatric nurses spent more time in hospital and day-care and had more out-patient attendances when compared to the control group. Whether this is considered 'inferior' is a value judgment. One could assert that contact with community psychiatric nurses could be leading to early detection of crises and treatment of problems (as evidenced by increased time in hospital care). This could be perceived as preferable by patient and family. The differences in admission may not be related to community psychiatric nursing care at all, but to other variables, for example better prognosis or family support; this would support Mangen and Griffith's comment that matching may have been inadequate.

Hunter's study, nevertheless, provided valuable information about the outcome and process of community psychiatric nursing. He found that the most disturbed patients (as judged by the carers) were not receiving community psychiatric nursing care. This may suggest that the community psychiatric nurses' contribution leads to less disturbance in patients whom they visit, or that it increases relatives' tolerance and ability to cope with the disturbance. Hunter also found that patients' families do not seek help when they need it. He concluded that less stress should be placed on one-to-one relationships between nurses and patients, and that more emphasis should be placed on social relationships and the development of interpersonal skills.

Hunter provided little information on the methods of data collection. He suggested that he gained information from records (1978, p.77), but it is unclear which records were being referred to. The 'in-depth' detail of information suggests that structured interviews may have been used by the nurses and researcher, but reference is made only to research interviews (1978, p.58) and the fact that 'nurses described their work' (1978, p.62–3). Hunter provided a case study format and compared nurse–patient–carer comments about patient care; this was combined with the researcher's analysis of the work of community psychiatric nurses. He, therefore, provided consumer feedback about the value of the community psychiatric nursing service to families with schizophrenic relatives.

Studies which use patient samples composed of subjects already referred to community psychiatric nurses may be biased towards individuals thought to be at relatively higher risk of relapse. Paykel and his colleagues (1982, 1983), to avoid this bias which was present in Hunter's study, used a prospective randomised clinical trial. This study compared community psychiatric nursing care of a group of chronically neurotic women with the outpatient care from psychiatrists. Undertaken over an 18-month period, this study used many measures of outcome: symptoms; social functioning; family burden; consumer satisfaction; and economic cost.

The authors demonstrated that the community psychiatric nurses did equally as well as psychiatrists. The community psychiatric nurses were, in fact, perceived as being 'warmer', and patients were more satisfied with this care. This study also provided information about the 'process' of community psychiatric nursing: community psychiatric nurses followed up the patients for longer than did the psychiatrists, and this follow-up was systematic, in that discharge was planned, with gradual reduction of frequency of visits. Community psychiatric nursing care achieved more discharges by the end of the 18-month study period than was achieved by the doctors. There was a small increase in the number of GP contacts among the community psychiatric nurse/patient group.

The limitation of both of these outcome studies is that they focus on specific diagnostic categories of patients, and the findings are not necessarily generalisable to all patients cared for by community psychiatric nurses. A recent study by Rushforth (1986), focusing on parasuicide patients cared for by community psychiatric nurses, continues this emphasis.

Marks (1985) conducted a randomised, year-long clinical trial, also on neurotic patients, but comparing treatment by nurse therapists (psychiatric nurses with an additional behaviour therapy training) with care by GPs. Brooker (1985b) compared community psychiatric nurses with nurse therapists and commented that the main difference between the two was that therapists had a skills-based training. It is not known to what extent this training affects patient care as no research has been completed comparing the work of the community psychiatric nurse and nurse therapist. In Marks' study, patients who received treatment from nurse therapists did better when compared with the GP group. At the end of one year, control patients who had not improved had crossover behavioural treatment, and they then improved. The author indicated the worthwhile gains that might ensue for patients and community from psychiatric nurses assuming a greater role in the care of patients with neuroses. It was suggested that GPs sought the advice of the nurses about general psychiatric patients, hence extending the nurse's role to 'that of a community psychiatric nurse' (Marks, 1985, p.1183). The measures used by Marks were problem- and leisure-ratings, problem-related targets and a self-administered fear questionnaire; no assessment of family burden was attempted. This study also focused on a narrowly defined group of patients.

Relevance of literature review to the study

Structure
The above review of the literature on community psychiatric nursing services shows that evaluation research has taken place on a limited basis. There is a lack of information on community psychiatric nursing at the 'structural' level. Repetition of the CPNA Survey of 1985 and implementation of the DHSS Korner Recommendations (see p.61) will rectify this to a certain extent.

Process
There is also a lack of evaluative research focusing on the 'process' of community psychiatric nursing; overall, to date, this has been in quantitative terms, and there is a need for more information which generates 'qualitative' detail on the work of the community psychiatric nurse. McKendrick (1980) commented, 'Decisions are made daily on the organisation and development of community psychiatric nursing services throughout the country and little is known of the criteria upon which such decisions are based'. The present study attempts to fill in this gap and provides some answers to McKendrick's statement.

Outcome
Outcome studies on community psychiatric nursing are few; those which have been undertaken have been on specific diagnostic categories of patients (neurotics and schizophrenics) and have tended to use researcher-orientated measures of outcome. There is a need to evaluate 'outcomes' in relation to other diagnostic groups for whom community psychiatric nurses care. This factor underpinned

the decisions relating to sample choice in the present study. There also appears to be a lack of information linking process with outcome, and this, too, was a focus of interest in the present study.

THE GOALS AND OBJECTIVES OF COMMUNITY PSYCHIATRIC NURSING

Introduction

In reviewing the current policy documents on provision of psychiatric care, it was found that there was a lack of elaboration of strategy towards defined goals. The next section of the literature review explores whether or not this is also the case for community psychiatric nursing. The goals and objectives of community psychiatric nursing are elaborated, and the reasons for choosing the carer as the focus of interest in this study are given.

Strategy and community psychiatric nursing
The lack of elaboration of strategy towards defined goals, evident in policy documents, raised questions about whether this is also the case for community psychiatric nursing. Use of the word 'strategy' suggests a plan or method (the term has military derivations which include 'the art of manoeuvring an army effectively' and 'a large scale plan for winning a war'). By implication, plans have objectives and goals.

Review of the community psychiatric nursing literature provides evidence that authors are searching for 'explanations' of service development rather than citing evidence of planning towards achievable goals. Many of the descriptions provided do not mention any theoretical framework surrounding community psychiatric nursing service development, and much of the information provided is anecdotal (Ainsworth and Jolley, 1978; Brennan, 1981; Sencicle, 1981).

Reasons for the development of community psychiatric nursing
Reasons for service development seem to be stated in preference to highlighting goals. The 'reasons' given include various expressed purposes or intentions, recommended/prescribed tasks and perceived advantages. These illustrate the ambiguity of the word 'reason' but yield information about implicit goals, objectives and 'process' criteria.

The reasons for the development of community psychiatric nursing reflect two different levels of argument, one arguing for the development of community psychiatric nursing, and the other arguing at the level of why specific services have developed. Often rationales are not separated clearly. The confusion discussed earlier in relation to community care at the conceptual level is mirrored here.

An examination of accounts of service development reveals a number of different types of rationale, some having quite complex ramifications, variations and structures. A typology of the rationales behind community psychiatric nursing service development is listed numerically below. It shows that the stimulus for development has come from desires to improve the organisation of services to patients, hence improving patient care (rationales 1–4, 6 and 8 below), to improve the family's coping capacity (rationales 7 and 8), to improve interprofessional relationships (rationale 5), to improve psychiatric nursing itself (rationales 10, 11 and 12), and for economic reasons (rationale 9).

Diverse motivations have spurred the development of community psychiatric nursing: local factors, presence or absence of professionals and willingness of other professionals to collaborate, combined with theoretical discussion of the preference of community care to institutional care, have given an impetus to community psychiatric nursing in specific areas.

The rationales

1. Institutional care leads to secondary handicap which is considered undesirable and it is, therefore, argued that patients should not be admitted to hospital but preferably nursed at home (Roberts, 1976).

2. In accordance with government policy (and current professional practice), there is a desire to reduce the numbers of inpatients and the length of hospital stay (MacDonald, 1972). Pressure on hospital beds requires early discharge to vacate beds (MacDonald, 1972; Sharpe, 1975). There is evidence in the literature that discharge can result in 'the revolving door syndrome', where a pattern of short-term treatment and early discharge becomes repetitive. Nurses were, therefore, commissioned to undertake a supervisory and aftercare service (Kirkpatrick, 1967; Willey, 1969; Nickerson, 1972; Sharpe, 1975; Marais, 1976); to try to avoid this relapse pattern. Psychiatric nurses were considered the ideal group to assume this role by providing 'continuity' from hospital care and by using the developing relationship to effect change (Kirkpatrick, 1967; Warren, 1971).

3. Community care, that is nursing of the patient outside the hospital, is preferred to institutional care as patients can avoid being labelled (Shires, 1977; Cohen, 1978; Jeevendrampillai, 1982). Stobie and Hopkins (1972a,b) talk of avoiding the crisis of admission, and Harker et al (1976) comment that contact with community psychiatric nurses avoids stigma. It is argued that care outside hospital can allow

patients to maintain their role for as long as possible (Stobie and Hopkins, 1972a,b), and responsibility can be maintained within the social group of the family (Ritson, 1977; Pullen and Gilbert, 1979a).

4.   The availability of drugs, particularly the long-acting preparations of phenothiazines, is considered effective in preventing relapse of patients, especially schizophrenic patients whose frequent readmissions were (assumed to be) related to failure to comply with drug regimes (Warren, 1971). Community psychiatric nurses were considered the most appropriate professionals to administer these drugs in the home situation (Warren, 1971; Nickerson, 1972; Leopoldt, 1974).

5.   Implicit in the literature is the suggestion that community psychiatric nurses can influence and change the attitudes of professionals and the public (MacDonald, 1972; Stobie and Hopkins, 1972a,b; Sharpe, 1980; Higgins, 1984). Psychiatric nurses possess particular skills (Kirkpatrick, 1967; Haque, 1973) which are transferable and useful in the community setting. Roberts (1976) has commented that community psychiatric nurses can act in a consultative capacity to non-psychiatric nurses who may have problems dealing with people showing symptoms of mental disorder. Clarke (1980) used research evidence on psychiatric morbidity to argue that community psychiatric nurse and health visitor liaison is needed. Anderson (1972) has commented on the need for community psychiatric nurses to educate other professionals with regard to psychiatric knowledge.

6.   Assessment at home, by the community psychiatric nurse, enables contact with relatives and, accordingly, can give greater insight into a patient's behaviour (Stobie and Hopkins, 1972a; Henderson et al, 1973; Hunter, 1978) and provide supplementary information on social history and living situations (May, 1965a,b; Weeks and Greene, 1966).

7.   Home assessment also enables community psychiatric nurses to offer support to the family and carers of the patient (Barker and Black, 1971; Roberts, 1976).

8.   Community psychiatric nurses can implement treatment quickly and early help can be given which helps both patients and carers (MacDonald, 1972, Leopoldt, 1979a, b).

9.   Community psychiatric nurses can relieve medical-staff time at outpatient clinics (Leopoldt, 1973; Sharpe, 1975), and they can see patients previously dealt with by a psychiatrist (Leopoldt, 1975) or can compensate for a shortage of psychiatric social workers (Sharpe, 1975).

Three other reasons have been given to justify the continued development of community psychiatric nursing.

10.   The work of the community psychiatric nurse is considered to be rewarding and interesting, and may involve learning new skills (Henderson et al, 1973), increased job satisfaction (Maisey, 1975), and reduction in the wastage of psychiatric nurses (MacDonald, 1972).

11.   Experience provided by community psychiatric nursing teams was considered beneficial to students and trained nurses whose training was considered to be too institutionally orientated (Sharpe, 1975).

12.   Community psychiatric nurses were considered to fulfil a useful function as disseminators of information to the team and institution on family and social aspects (Maisey, 1975).

As can be seen from this list, most of the writing about reasons for development took place in the 1970s. This seems to have coincided with a marked increase in the number of CPNs and interest in the speciality of community psychiatric nursing; documentation of 'reasons' for development may be linked to the need for the speciality to gain recognition. Since the 1970s, community psychiatric nursing has gained acceptance within the field and the literature of the '80s has moved on from general comments about the reasons why community psychiatric nurses are needed, to looking at more specific issues like education and training, details about practice and evaluation of the effectiveness of services.

Goal-setting and community psychiatric nursing

Community psychiatric nursing services do not seem to set goals for their corporate activities, although individual nurses are increasingly using a systematic approach to care. Recent papers, for instance, suggest that goal-setting is a feature of community psychiatric nurses' work with individual patients (Ditton, 1984; Persaud, 1985). This is related to the increased use of 'nursing process' approaches to patient care taken by some community psychiatric nurses (Williamson, 1982). Goal-setting otherwise does not appear to be a feature of the work of community psychiatric nursing services. Goals can be inferred from the reasons given, but authors tend not to elaborate on these, nor to examine whether specific aims are met.

Statistical data, although not entirely satisfactory as a means of evaluation of services, may be utilised to ascertain goal attainment. Inasmuch as one can make general comments based on the literature, descriptive statistics on community psychiatric nursing services appear to be collected routinely, analysed retrospectively and used to justify changes in the patterns of community psychiatric nursing care rather than for forward planning (Maisey, 1975; Leopoldt, 1979a,b; Sharpe, 1980). Only two articles provide evidence of statistics being used for forward planning, those of Sharpe (1982) and Holloway

(1984). Sharpe (1982) conducted a survey of GPs in the Croydon area in order to plan a future community psychiatric nursing service. He found that 84% of the GPs wanted an attached community psychiatric nurse, and he was able to gain a clear idea of these GPs' expectations of such a nurse. Holloway (1984) carried out a project which demonstrated the value of a proposed mental health centre and resulted in improvement and changes in future service provision.

These two papers could be the tip of a large, hidden iceberg, of course, but the lack of statistics at national level (see. p.61) would give some support to the conclusion that statistics are not used for planning services. The present study looks at the goals set by two community psychiatric nursing services and investigates the work of community psychiatric nursing to examine the values and assumptions underpinning the work at local level.

The literature and contact with carers

Three of the above-listed reasons for development of the service refer to the carers of the mentally ill and state the advantages of community psychiatric nurse contact with carers. Contact between the nurses and carers is considered to be beneficial to the nurses and to facilitate the process of assessment and treatment of patients. (By implication, this will also help the patients and carers, as appropriate and speedy care will be implemented.) Community psychiatric nursing contact is also considered beneficial to the carers, who, it is argued, receive support and also relief at the earliest opportunity.

The discussion above on the effect of community care policies suggests that the 'family' (especially female kin) are expected to look after sick members, and that this expectation shows little sign of changing. In view of this, it seems appropriate to take stock of the present situation and assess what support carers are currently receiving.

Obviously, carers could receive 'support' from a variety of sources (see Blaxter, 1976, and Orford, 1987, for a summary of the issues involved). The above comments indicate, however, that 'support of the carers' is one reason for the existence of the community psychiatric nursing service. This study was, therefore, intended to assess the help which carers perceive as being given by community psychiatric nurses. Furthermore, this study provided the opportunity to examine the process of community psychiatric nursing and find out to what extent supporting the carers affected the work of community psychiatric nurses.

A brief review of the literature pertaining to community psychiatric nurses' contact with carers follows.

There have been two trains of thought as regards the family and the work of the community psychiatric nurse, and these have differentiated even the first two community psychiatric nursing services which were developed. At Warlingham Park Hospital, May and Moore (1963) commented:

'... detailed investigation of the patient's family situation or modification of his environment and of difficulties in interpersonal relationships is not expected.'

Community psychiatric nursing work in the above-mentioned community psychiatric nursing service was closely supervised by a consultant psychiatrist. Clearly, this service did not expect therapeutic change by the involvement of community psychiatric nurses in family work, although it was acknowledged that community psychiatric nurses would reassure relatives by their continued contact.

The other early community psychiatric nursing service at Moorhaven Hospital (Weeks and Greene, 1966), in contrast, recognised that community psychiatric nurses would have an active role with the family. This service, supervised by a social worker considered knowledgeable in family care, developed with the expressed aim that community psychiatric nurses should look for stresses within the family and take appropriate steps to remedy these (Llewelyn, 1974).

These two services have very different focuses of attention. The first has a primary focus on the patient who is considered to be 'separate' from the social network in which he lives. Other services have developed like this, in which the family is only considered as being peripherally important to the patient. Sharpe (1975), for example, cites 13 reasons for the work of community psychiatric nurses; only one of these makes reference to relatives. The second focus is one in which the family is viewed as an integral part of patient care. These two approaches are comparable to using the medical model and social model of care respectively. Using the former model, a person becomes a passive patient where behaviour is observed and 'symptoms' are isolated and treated; using a social model of care, the patient is seen as actively involved in a social network which is included in the care given.

Studies of psychiatric nurses' work in the hospital setting suggest that nurses are minimally involved with relatives. Cormack (1976) found that, in the hospital setting, psychiatric nurses were rarely seen to initiate conversations with patients' relatives; only 2% of nursing activities involved relatives. These were similar findings to those of Oppenheim and Eeman (1955). Cormack also found that contacts with relatives were held in a public place, that patients were rarely present and that the content of the interactions was related to superficial information exchange rather than to the participation of the relatives as part of the treatment process.

It is reasonable to assume that, compared with hospital- or ward-based psychiatric nurses, community psychiatric nurses may be involved more with relatives. Because community psychiatric nurses are providing care in the home situation, contact with carers is more likely to occur than it is in psychiatric hospitals which are typically situated in inaccessible rural settings. To visit patients in their own home situation is different: in the patient's home, the nurse is the guest and the dynamics are different. One would assume too that, by virtue of the family's involvement in caring, the family, patient and community psychiatric nurse would all, by necessity, be actively involved.

Do community psychiatric nurses have contact with relatives in the home situation? This, of course, depends in the first instance on whether the relatives live with the patients. Quine (1981) has shown that many discharged patients do not live with relatives. Harrison (1984) found that almost half of the patients in a community psychiatric nursing sample had no relatives living nearby. It could be that community psychiatric nurses tend to visit patients without families. The patients of the community psychiatric nurses in Harrison's study (1984) were elderly – availability of relatives may depend on patient type. Creer et al (1982) found that, even after many years of illness, as many as 50% of patients may still be in contact with relatives.

If relatives are available, do community psychiatric nurses interact with them? Available evidence is inconsistent. Skidmore and Friend (1984a) found that few community psychiatric nurses interacted at all with relatives. Pullen (1980), however, described an extramural psychiatric service and commented that, in one third of home visits, involvement of relatives was 'useful', although no elaboration of 'useful for what' was provided. He commented that 80% of the visits included contact with the relatives; this was compared with only 17% of the outpatient attenders. Sladden (1979) showed that relatives were seen with 2% of patients who attended an injection clinic, but were present in 40% of the home visits. Thus, compared with outpatient appointments, home care allows contact with the family, and the setting in which patients are seen may be an important influence on whether or not relatives are also seen by the community psychiatric nurses.

Sladden also analysed nurse/patient contacts; she found that observation and assessment activities were more numerous if a family member was present. This suggests that relatives are involved in the assessment activities of the community psychiatric nurses rather than in treatment. Sladden found that community psychiatric nurses used cognitive approaches to patients and families. These were more frequently used at initial contacts and especially where patients were deteriorating. The community psychiatric nurses in the study only appeared actively to help patients and families to understand the situation in times of crisis; helping patients and families gain under-standing of the situation was not seen as ongoing work.

Sladden's findings showed that family members (if present) provided information that was helpful to community psychiatric nurses in assessment, but that they did not take up the opportunity of these contacts in long-term therapy. No information was gained in this study about the family's view of the service (an omission fully acknowledged by the researcher herself). There, indeed, seems to be a need to gain information from the family about the benefits of community psychiatric nursing contact, in order to assess accurately whether or not community psychiatric nurses should involve families in treatment. This was explored in the present study.

The literature and 'burden'

One of the reasons underlying the work of the community psychiatric nurses with carers was to help them to cope with caring for a mentally-ill relative at home. What evidence is there in the literature that the carers need help?

One of the major effects of the change in orientation of care (i.e. from institutional care to care in the community) is that patients spend less time in hospital and more time with the people with whom they live, often the family. Several authors have provided evidence of the effect that the presence of a mentally-ill person can have on relatives. Kreitman (1964) showed, in a controlled study, that spouses of neurotic patients have more physical and psychological symptoms than normal control subjects. Other studies have since showed that families are affected in many ways by other types of chronic mental illness (Wing et al, 1964; Waters and Northover, 1965; Rutter, 1966).

This effect on families is loosely described in the literature as 'burden', a term coined by Grad and Sainsbury (1963, 1968). A widespread interest was shown in the topic of 'burden' in the 1960s, when community care programmes were enthusiastically intro-duced. Since then, schizophrenic patients constitute the only group in which interest in family burden has been sustained. A recent chapter by Kuipers (1987), which reviews the effect of depression on family life, and publications by Gilhooly (1984) and Scottish Action on Dementia (1986a,b), suggest that interest in the relationship of 'burden' to other mental illnesses may be reviving. Kreisman and Joy (1974), nevertheless, criticised researchers for taking a 'scatter-shot' approach to their data, and for failing to follow through on promising leads; they commented, 'This lack of sustained interest has left us with fundamental pieces of information missing'.

The features of 'burden' have more often been commented on than objectively studied (Willey, 1969; Ashton, 1978; Moore, 1982;

Eastwood, 1983). The dissection of the concept of burden through its effects on the performance of various roles fulfilled by the patient's relatives was an approach first taken by Mills (1962). The study of Grad and Sainsbury (1963, 1968) advanced the measurement of 'burden' by using a three-point rating scale rather than the descriptive sketches given by their predecessors. These authors showed that caring for a psychiatrically-ill relative could cause disturbance in the social and leisure activities of families, disturb the domestic routine, upset other members of the household, affect their capacity to work by making demands and obstructing employment opportunities, and strain the mental and physical health of the carers.

Hoenig and Hamilton (1967, 1969) also investigated burden. They differentiated between 'objective' burden (the severity of difficulty observed) and 'subjective' burden (the degree of strain reported). They found a disparity between the two types of burden. The meaning of this disparity is unclear, but it was interpreted by Hoenig and Hamilton as evidence of the willingness on the part of relatives to assume a burden. As Hoenig and Hamilton point out, 'A burden may be taken on in loving care and as a source of obligation and not sensed as such and may be preferred to what others, anxious to help, regard as relief'. This disparity may, however, be evidence of relatives' reluctance to complain about caring or relatives' low expectation of service provision (Hawks, 1975).

In Hoenig and Hamilton's study, 46% of families felt that the patient was a burden; 75% of these did not complain although they were suffering severe objective and subjective burden. Grad and Sainsbury found that many relatives had suffered problems for more than two years. Hunter (1978) found that schizophrenic patients' relatives did not ask community psychiatric nurses for help even if they needed it. These studies and others (Creer and Wing, 1974; Creer et al, 1982) strongly suggest that many relatives will not ask for help and that, if service provision is based on demands from relatives, lengthy periods of suffering will be experienced before help is given. Furthermore, these authors drew clear inferences from their findings for future service provision, which were aimed at helping families to cope and at providing community facilities to relieve carers. The failure of the mental health service professionals to do this is well documented (see Creer et al, 1982). Recent studies do, however, suggest that professional intervention with families caring for schizophrenic patients is being undertaken on a limited basis, and that this is beneficial to patients and carers (Falloon et al, 1982; Leff et al, 1982; Barrowclough and Tarrier, 1984; Tarrier and Barrowclough, 1986).

Burden should not necessarily be presumed to be a negative experience undergone reluctantly. Studies of carers' experiences have revealed evidence of carers benefiting from living with a psychiatrically-ill relative. Stevens (1972) described how tolerance of a patient is not necessarily dysfunctional, but can lead to social solidarity of the family and prevent social isolation of elderly relatives.

The weight of opinion, however, is that negative effects and disruption of family life are caused by caring for a psychiatrically-ill dependent (Creer and Wing, 1974; Pai and Kapur, 1982; Pai and Nagarajaiah, 1982; Gibbons et al, 1984). The Equal Opportunities Reports (Equal Opportunities Commission, 1980, 1982a,b, 1984) also reveal a picture of employment and social opportunities foregone, physical fatigue and emotional stress, all compounded by financial difficulties and lack of social recognition. These surveys focused on carers of elderly and handicapped relatives. Other authors have drawn similar conclusions: Wheatley (1980a, b) in a study focusing on care of the elderly, Wertheimer (1982) and Bayley (1973) in relation to care of the mentally handicapped, and Topliss and Gould (1981) and Blaxter (1976) as regards the physically handicapped.

As Blaxter (1976) has commented, families have to cope with many crises and adjust their life-style to accommodate changing circumstances of family members: poverty or unemployment, someone leaving by marriage, emigration, or death, prison sentences or new jobs are but a few possible examples of change. It is unclear from the literature whether the mechanisms required to cope with these life events are similar to those required to care for a dependent relative. It is also unclear whether different stresses are involved in caring for a mentally- or physically-ill relative, or what different stresses are associated with different diagnostic categories.

Accounts given of carers' experiences suggest that the negative effects of mental illness are the most burdensome: Creer and Wing (1974) found that withdrawal such as lack of conversation, under-activity and slowness were problematic for relatives; Vaughn and Leff (1976a,b) found that lack of communication, interest, affection and initiative were the focus of the majority of critical comments made by relatives; Fadden et al (1987) found that the negative symptoms of depressive illness were the most difficult to deal with. Grad and Sainsbury's studies (1963, 1968) showed that the relatives most burdened were those caring for patients with organic psychosis, suggesting that the combination of physical sequelae with mental illness is particularily stressful.

The literature reviewed above suggests that there are legitimate reasons for community psychiatric nurses' contact with relatives if they can help them cope with 'burden'.

The literature and schizophrenia

In addition to helping carers to cope with 'burden', the literature suggests that community psychiatric nurses could help the families of schizophrenic patients in other ways. As far as schizophrenic patients are concerned, contact with the family plays a crucial role in the course of the illness.

Early studies of discharged schizophrenic patients suggested that 'with whom' the patient lived seemed to influence the course of the illness. Brown et al (1958) followed up 229 male patients on discharge from hospital. They found that successful outcome was associated with patients' clinical state on discharge, with their subsequent employment, and with the social group into which they were discharged. Patients staying with parents, wives or in large hostels did *less* well than those staying with siblings or in lodgings. The findings also suggested that there was an optimum degree of stimulation which suited schizophrenic patients; what the relatives did (or did not do – see below) influenced the course of schizophrenia.

Brown's initial observations were further extended in a series of increasingly elaborate studies (Brown et al, 1962, 1966, 1972; Rutter, 1966; Vaughn and Leff, 1976a,b). These strongly suggested that it was not the relationship between the carer and the patient that affected the course of schizophrenia but, rather, the behaviour of the key relative.

Leff and Vaughn have coined the term 'expressed emotion', to describe this behaviour (Leff and Vaughn, 1976a,b); this is a measure of the number of critical comments made by relatives and the extent of emotional overinvolvement and hostility expressed within the family (as assessed by use of the Camberwell Family Interview). They noted that certain families with a schizophrenic member demonstrated 'high expressed emotion', and that patients returning to live with these relatives had a higher relapse rate than those returning to 'low expressed emotion' families. Recent evidence suggests that this factor may also be relevant to depressed patients (see Hooley et al, 1986).

There appear to be two ways of minimising this effect. Leff and Vaughn (1981) suggested that medication might have a protective effect on schizophrenic patients who lived with 'high expressed emotion' families. They further suggested (1976a) that reducing contact with relatives, to less than 35 hours per week, had a protective effect on these patients.

Barrowclough and Tarrier (1984) reviewed the studies assessing the effect of psychosocial interventions with schizophrenic families and considered the studies of Leff et al (1982) and Falloon et al (1982) to be well designed. The results indicate the benefit to families, of (social) intervention, which can reduce the incidence of relapse of schizophrenic illness.

Leff et al (1982) prospectively allocated 'high expressed emotion' patient/families to differing treatment groups, either routine outpatient treatment or intervention aimed at helping families to reduce the number of critical comments and face-to-face contacts with patients. A follow-up study has since been completed with similar results (Leff et al, 1985). Falloon et al's study (1982) allocated schizophrenics on maintenance medication to either home treatment or clinic-based supportive care. The family therapy approach sought to lessen stress in the patient and family through improved understanding of the illness and through behavioural training to problem solving. After nine months, the family approach to treatment was seen to be clearly superior.

This section clearly demonstrates the interventions that are possible for families looking after schizophrenic relatives and indicates that community psychiatric nurses could have a valid role to play with carers.

The literature and continuity

Before ending this section, it is worth discussing the notion of 'continuity of care'. This is relevant to the care given to carers by community psychiatric nurses.

Community psychiatric nurses are assumed to provide 'continuity of care' to patients. Definition of the phrase 'continuity of care' is unclear. There seems to be a range of implied meanings covered by the term. Kirkpatrick (1967) suggests that 'continuity of care' means contact with the same nurse during and after hospitalisation, while Altschul (1972a, 1973) and Pullen (1980) use the term 'follow-up' to describe the implementation of a consistent treatment plan; the terms 'follow-up' and 'continuity of care' seem to be used interchangeably. Hunter (1974, 1978) describes community psychiatric nursing as providing a 'continuing care service'.

The idea behind 'continuity of care' seems to be that it is beneficial for patients to continue contact with psychiatric personnel who can provide on-going support to individuals and families (Hunter, 1974). Research which examined the effect of intervention with schizophrenic patients and their families (Falloon et al, 1982; Leff et al, 1982), and research which has studied the benefits of day care (Herz et al, 1971; Washburn et al, 1976), lends support to this claim.

Hunter (1978) furnishes us with information on patients' and families' feelings about 'continuity of care'. He reported that the care-givers appreciated the long-term support of the community psychiatric nurses. However, he found that the emphasis of care was on the patient, and he recommended that 'more active and open co-operation should be sought from care-givers in particular'.

Allied to the notion of 'continuity of care' is the belief that it is wrong to discharge patients, either to a non-psychiatric professional or to no professional care at all, after an acute phase of illness or after a long period of hospitalisation (Ashton, 1978). This belief has been encouraged by the recent literature which suggests that community care policies result in patients being 'dumped' in bedsitters and doss houses and generally neglected by the psychiatric services (McBrien, 1985; Brown, 1985b). Sladden (1979) found that the nurses in her study tended to keep patients on the books and were reluctant to discharge them. This 'holding on' to patients could be interpreted as reflecting the community psychiatric nurses' fear of public or professional criticism.

Also implied in the term 'continuity of care' is that a relationship between patient and nurse is continuing to develop (Kirkpatrick, 1967; Hunter, 1974). Paykel et al (1982, 1983) provided some research evidence to support the idea that relationships develop between patients and nurses. These authors found that community psychiatric nurses were perceived by patients as being 'warmer' than were doctors visited on an outpatient basis. The patients were also more satisfied with the care received, suggesting that patients make judgments about the quality of the relationships they have with their therapists (although this could also suggest that patients do not want to make the effort to travel to outpatient departments!).

It is unclear whether tasks need to be undertaken to ensure that a relationship develops between nurse and patient. Hunter (1978) found that injection-giving led to conversation between the nurse/patient/care-giver stopping. It is also unclear whether a relationship with one individual nurse is desirable and necessary to provide 'continuity of care'. Sladden (1979) found that many patients had contact with either *one* community psychiatric nurse (these patients were usually seen in the home situation) or *all five* community psychiatric nurses in the study (most of whom were seen in the injection clinic).

The term 'continuity of care' is also used to refer to contacts with other professionals and agencies with whom the community psychiatric nurse and patient have contact. Other authors use different terms for this activity, e.g. liaison, but the implication is that this activity is needed to provide continued care to patients. Sladden (1979) found that the community psychiatric nurses did not value contacts with GPs, and Hunter (1978) found that there was little contact between community psychiatric nurses and other agencies.

Examination of the term 'continuity of care' has shown that understanding of the term is varied and confused and that the research evidence which is available on community psychiatric nursing and 'continuity of care' is limited. Examination of the nurses' work will allow exploration of whether or not this is a relevant concept for the community psychiatric nurses.

In this section, the goals inherent in the work of community psychiatric nursing have been examined, and, in particular, the nurse's work with carers has been focused on. This leads to the choice of the 'carer' as one of the major foci of this study, and emphasises the need to examine the work of the community psychiatric nurses.

To summarise, the 'carer' is chosen as the focus for several reasons. First, some of the documented rationales given for community psychiatric nursing service provision include giving support and help to the carers of the mentally ill who are looked after at home. The literature further confirms that community psychiatric nurses could have a legitimate role with relatives either by specific interventions to reduce the 'burden' or 'expressed emotion' experienced by carers, or by providing continuity of care.

Secondly, review of the literature on community-care policies suggests that the 'family', especially women, care for the mentally ill at home. In view of this and the limited 'community' resources available, it seems timely, therefore, to find out what support carers are currently receiving from the community psychiatric nursing services. This, combined with the burdensome (seriously onerous and negative) nature of the carers' experiences, underlines the importance of evaluating the effect of the community psychiatric nursing input.

Finally, there has been little recent interest in the topic of 'burden'; this appears to be an omission if one considers the fact that the role of family and non-professionals in care of the mentally ill seems to be on the increase. These comments indicate that it is urgent to attempt an evaluation of the help received by informal carers.

The present study examines carers' perceptions of help received from community psychiatric nurses. Examination of the process of community psychiatric nursing will show how 'supporting the carers' is viewed by nurses.

THE NATIONAL CONTEXT OF THE STUDY

The following section presents a brief historical review of the development of community psychiatric nursing services and sets the national framework within which the present study was completed. Review of the literature in this section confirmed the decision to focus the study on examination of the work of community psychiatric nursing itself and suggested an investigation of a service at local level.

To summarise what follows: the relevant policy documents are examined and these show that the evolution of community psychiatric nursing services has been unplanned at national level, and that, as a result, community psychiatric nursing services lack shared, explicit policies.

There is uncertainty about how staffing levels for community psychiatric services should be decided. Manpower data for community psychiatric nursing are either unavailable or are concealed within national/regional and local data for psychiatric nursing in general. The Korner Recommendations could (although not being adopted in Scotland) offer an alternative model to change this situation (Department of Health and Social Security, 1984).

Any prescription or data-base must contain presuppositions about aims, goals and objectives of community psychiatric nursing. As we saw in the previous section, which explored the goals and objectives of the community psychiatric nursing services, there are few accurate descriptions about the work of community psychiatric nurses and there is uncertainty about what standards the service is aiming for or hoping to achieve. The following review shows that policy-makers recommend target figures for the development of community psychiatric nursing as a speciality. This would seem to be paradoxical when community psychiatric nurses' work is still not clearly defined. It seems illogical to recommend an increase in numbers of community psychiatric nurses when there is doubt about what they do.

Policy documents and speciality development

Community psychiatric nursing as a speciality has been gaining a higher profile over the years. The first recorded beginnings of community psychiatric nursing were in 1954 at Warlingham Park Hospital and in 1952 in Moorhaven Hospital (May and Moore, 1963; Greene, 1968). The first official document which discusses community psychiatric nursing (Department of Health and Social Security, 1975) called it 'a district psychiatric nursing service'. In 1968, only passing reference was made that community psychiatric nursing was worthy of 'general study' (Ministry of Health Central Health Services Council, 1968). That community psychiatric nursing was developing during this period is borne out by Brook and Cooper (1975).

Because of the apparent increase of community psychiatric nurses, Parnell (1974) was commissioned to carry out the first survey of community psychiatric nursing in England and Wales. By 1980, community psychiatric nursing was sufficiently recognised within the mental health field to warrant the attention of psychiatrists (Royal College of Psychiatrists, 1980). In 1981, the Royal College of General Practitioners commented on the value of community psychiatric nursing intervention during crises and life changes (Royal College of General Practitioners, 1981). Recent policy documents have devoted considerable space to the discussion of community psychiatric nursing (Scottish Home and Health Department, 1985; Social Services Committee, 1985). However, despite the increased interest in, and assertions of, the 'general' value of community psychiatric nursing, policy documents are still unclear about what is offered by community psychiatric nurses and the services in which they work. It is not surprising, therefore, to find that the training needs of community psychiatric nurses are still being debated and argued; a prerequisite to the development of any training course must be the possession of a clear idea of what the nurses are being trained *for*. This clarity of purpose is absent in community psychiatric nursing today.

Training and community psychiatric nursing

Specific training for this role started in the early 1970s, but has been slow to expand and has still been received only by a minority of practising community psychiatric nurses.

In 1974, an outline curriculum for a community psychiatric nursing course (a post-registration course for registered mental nurses) was published (Leopoldt, 1974). Other courses have been mounted for the training of community psychiatric nurses: England has nine training centres for community psychiatric nursing, Scotland, three. The contents of these courses are difficult to define and are not as well described as other post-registration courses such as behaviour therapy (Brooker, 1985b). The courses offered have been criticised because they do not offer training in specific clinical skills (Brooker, 1984a; Skidmore and Friend, 1984b, Community Psychiatric Nurses Association, 1985a).

The number of trained community psychiatric nurses

Not all practising community psychiatric nurses, however, have undergone a post-registration course. Dunnel and Dobbs (1982) estimated that only about 15% of the community psychiatric nurses in their sample had completed courses in community psychiatric nursing. Brooker noted that this figure was an underestimate, and calculated (based on English National Board data) that only 725 out of the total of 2500 community psychiatric nurses in England were trained (Brooker, 1985b). Based on responses to parliamentary questions on trained community psychiatric nurses, there were 181 trained community psychiatric nurses in Scotland in 1983 (McKay, 1985). The Community Psychiatric Nurses Association conducted a survey of community psychiatric nurses in Scotland and England (Community Psychiatric Nurses Association, 1985b), which found that only 22.4% (i.e. 618) of practising community psychiatric nurses had completed a community psychiatric nursing course. The survey also found that, since 1980, there had been an increase of only 303 in the number of community psychiatric nurses holding the post-registration certificate, compared with an increase in psychiatric nurses working in the community from 1667 to 2758 over the same period.

The issue of mandatory training for community psychiatric nurses has been the subject of much recent debate (Devlin, 1984; Manchester, 1984; Skidmore and Friend, 1984b, Simmons and Brooker, 1986; Dexter and Morrall, 1987). The Royal College of Nursing, along with the CPNA, has recommended mandatory training for community psychiatric nurses (Royal College of Nursing, 1982a) but training for community psychiatric nursing has, so far, remained optional and is still not a prerequisite to practice.

Against this background of uncertainty about what community psychiatric nurses do, and debate about how they are prepared for the work, policy documents have, nevertheless, made recommendations about developments of the speciality of community psychiatric nursing.

Population ratios and community psychiatric nursing development

How are levels of community psychiatric nurse staffing decided? There seem to be two main methods of doing this, the first based on population ratios, and the second based on estimates of need. It was proposed, for example, that psychiatric nurse staffing should be related to 'the total needs of the population' (Department of Health and Social Security, 1975). This vague reference to a 'population' in the statement is confusing as it is unclear which population this refers to: Britain-wide, Scotland-wide or that of the local areas. The concept of 'need' is also notoriously difficult to define (Blaxter, 1976). Since 1975, attempts to meet the 'needs' of the population have been met by establishing psychiatric nurse targets in relation to population ratios. In 1975 in England, community psychiatric nurses were included with psychiatric nurse staffing:

> 'In the light of present and expected future numbers of psychiatric nurses, the DHSS is aiming at an initial target in each health district of a level of psychiatric nurse staffing of 85 per 100,000 population increasing gradually as resources permit to 100 nurses per 100,000 population. The present national average is in excess of 90 per 100,000, but they are not evenly distributed.' (Department of Health and Social Security, 1975)

In Scotland, community psychiatric nurse staffing is still not considered separately from psychiatric nursing generally, targets for which are based on inpatient bed occupancy (CANO, 1975; Scottish Home and Health Department, 1985). These guidelines provide a basis for nurse staffing levels in residential institutions but they may not provide a model for community psychiatric nursing.

There is comment in the literature about the development of community psychiatric nursing services on the basis of community psychiatric nurse (CPN)-to-population ratios. The first reference to CPN-to-population ratios was by Brook and Cooper (1975) who suggested a suitable ratio as being 1 CPN to 30 000 members of the population. The most recent reference is by Marks (1985), who suggested a ratio of 1:25 000. Carr et al (1980) derived a ratio of 1:15 000 with an anticipated target of 1:7500 in the long term. The Community Psychiatric Nurses Association proposed a target of 1 CPN for each 10 000 members of the population (Community Psychiatric Nurses Association, 1985). This figure has been adopted as a desired ratio for the development of community psychiatric nursing services in at least one part of the United Kingdom, in connection with a planned hospital closure (Friern and Claybury Hospitals in North East Thames Regional Authority).

This method of deciding community psychiatric establishments has been criticised on methodological grounds (Brook and Cooper, 1975) and on the basis that the ratios are unrealistic (Royal College of Psychiatrists, 1980; Rushforth, 1986). Mangen and Griffith (1982a) suggest that professional interests have introduced 'bias in the data':

'In the current absence of adequate data on staffing needs in the mental health services, there are few reliable guidelines on which to depend. Such guidelines as there are, are input-orientated, relying on arbitrary assumptions about levels of need for mental health care and a particular agency's ability to meet them. The pressure to promote the interests of the profession under review adds to the bias in the data.'

Despite these criticisms, the use of targets and ratios has stimulated debate about the development of community psychiatric nursing within the larger field of psychiatric nursing and mental health care.

Difficulties of the development of community psychiatric nursing
Plans to develop community psychiatric nursing seem to be put forward without examination of the resulting implications. One of the problems facing community psychiatric nursing, for instance, as a developing speciality, is the problem of developing a new speciality in psychiatric nursing, when psychiatric nursing itself suffers from inadequate numbers (Scottish Home and Health Department, 1980a, 1985; Mental Welfare Commission, 1981). This problem is compounded in Scotland, as the following quote suggests:

'Improved recruitment of mental nurses is impeded by the fact that there is a single functional budget for nurse training and the great majority of student nurses go into general nurse training programmes. This approach maintains a self perpetuating pattern of recruitment which discourages improvements and developments in standards of care within the psychiatric services.' (Scottish Home and Health Department, 1985)

Another problem is that the development of community services and community psychiatric nursing increases the demands on the existing pool of trained psychiatric nurses (see p.3).

Numbers of community psychiatric nurses
Community psychiatric nursing has been described as a 'burgeoning' speciality (Devlin, 1985), but there is little information available on the scale and nature of the work of community psychiatric nurses, or on community psychiatric nursing staff numbers and deployment, to support this assertion.

This absence of a quantitative data-base on community psychiatric nursing was focused on by Baxter (1984) who calculated the growth in the number of community psychiatric nurses in the United Kingdom by looking at the demand for community psychiatric nurses in the 'situations vacant' column of a nursing journal. This is not a reliable method of collecting information about the growth of community psychiatric nursing. The lack of numerical information on community psychiatric nurses was referred to as 'gaps in the Department's system of statistical returns' (Social Services Committee Report, 1985) and has been commented on in the literature by Brook and Cooper (1975), Power (1976) and Shore (1977).

Two surveys conducted by the CPNA (Community Psychiatric Nurses Association, 1981, 1985b) provide the only available quantitative baseline examining changes in the development and organisation of community psychiatric nursing. These surveys show that between 1981 and 1985, across all grades, the number of community psychiatric nurses in Great Britain increased by 65%. The 1985 Survey made an attempt to provide a statistical analysis of community psychiatric nursing, but is primarily focused on England and Wales. Figures for Scotland as a whole (Community Psychiatric Nurses Association, 1985b) show that Scotland's existing community psychiatric nursing teams are predominantly hospital-based and receive most of their referrals from psychiatrists.

Health boards in Scotland do not seem to collect figures on community psychiatric nursing on a consistent basis; those that are available (from John McKay, in written replies to parliamentary questions in January, 1985) provide figures for qualified nurses only up to 1983 (see Drucker, 1987).

Data collection procedures
In this era of cost effectiveness (Dimmock, 1985a–c), it would appear to be a matter of urgency to examine, at national level, the resources which are being applied to community psychiatric nursing activity. At present, there is no standardised data-base for community psychiatric nursing, although quantitative measures are most commonly used to record the work of community psychiatric nurses.

A standardised data-base would facilitate a broad examination of, and provide a basis for comparison of, the structure, organisation and development of different community psychiatric nursing services. The DHSS has been reviewing its data-collection system, and community health services, including community psychiatric nursing, are being given special consideration (Department of Health and Social Security, 1984).

This report (the Korner Report) recommends the collection of information which will facilitate the assessment of psychiatric care in the community and on a nationwide basis. Managers will be obliged, by systematic and periodic evaluation, to look at their objectives and functions. The report also makes a distinction between services to the community – defined as prevention or intervention which is provided as a matter of policy – and patient care in the community – services in response to individual demand for treatment or care. This provides a framework for and challenge to community psychiatric nurses to clarify their work.

Quantitative measures

Many authors have focused on the difficulties of 'quantifying' aspects of community psychiatric nursing. For instance, Leopoldt (1975) said, 'A survey form can never present a complete picture. Number of referrals says nothing about the nature of the referrals, frequency of the visits, the distances travelled or the results achieved'. Brough (1980) argued that community psychiatric nurses' case-loads are not a useful baseline for estimating work-load. Beard (1980) commented that numbers of case-loads do not serve as a meaningful measurement on which to determine clinical input, safe practice or forward planning. McKendrick (1981b) has commented, 'Client dependency and nursing activity are difficult to quantify and the fluid nature of the community psychiatric nurse/client interaction does not lend itself to simplistic interpretations such as "timing of a visit"'. Measures which focus exclusively on patient or domiciliary contacts can be criticised as they take no account of the other activities of community psychiatric nurses, e.g. liaison with other professionals. Number of referrals and discharge rates do not simply equate with effectiveness. Clients' needs and team-functioning have to be considered.

Tyrell (1975) has commented that numbers have advantages in providing information to guide the use of resources, stating that they are less ambiguous than words alone and that they enable aspects of a situation to be seen in overall perspective. He warns that preferences or assumptions about the relevance of the measurement to the situation are always involved. The above authors would not support Tyrell's comments.

The current methods used to collect information on community psychiatric nursing are limited and have not been adapted to reflect the increase in psychiatric domiciliary work (Tyrell, 1975; Wiseman, 1981; McKendrick, 1981b). McKendrick examined the recording systems of a sample of community psychiatric nursing services and found that there was concern to measure the activities of the community psychiatric nurses at local level, but that there was little consensus (between services) as to which aspects of the community psychiatric nurses' work were important. McKendrick said, 'The initiatives of the community psychiatric nurses and community psychiatric nursing managers in introducing these measures of their performance is to be applauded ... as a method of evaluating and planning service'. Without accurate information about either the numbers or types of nursing personnel in community psychiatric nursing, or the quality of care provided, planning is difficult.

Planned development of community psychiatric nursing
Community psychiatric nursing appears to be developing rather haphazardly instead of in a planned and organised fashion. This is borne out by the comments of Mangen and Griffith (1982a):

> 'Community Psychiatric Nursing shares with other British social and health services a common history of isolated experimental development leading incrementally and without the benefit of clear policy guidelines to a national provision ... there is a great diversity in the range of patients managed in the therapeutic settings and in the forms of intervention.'

Numerical information supporting this 'local and uneven development' has only recently been available from the CPNA (Community Psychiatric Nurses Association, 1985b). The findings showed that:

> 'Community psychiatric nursing team growth is not correlated with population increase or decrease (OPCS 1985); an index of social deprivation (Rice et al 1985); or progress towards achieving Resource Allocation Working Party targets (Health Care, UK 1985).'

There remains a lack of information on community psychiatric nursing service development in Scotland (see above). Reasons for differing development in different areas are unclear. Brooker (1985a) interviewed a sample of managers in an attempt to find the reasons for community psychiatric nursing service development (or otherwise). He found that one of the reasons, related to growth, was that resulting from opportunities provided by joint funding which enabled increase of community psychiatric nursing teams.

Mangen and Griffith criticise the uneven development of community psychiatric nursing services: 'The local and ad hoc character of the development of services has given rise to serious problems in formulating an overall strategy' (Mangen and Griffith, 1982). The difficulties involved in formulating overall strategies for community psychiatric nursing mirror those of defining 'community care'.

The development of local community psychiatric nursing service
It could be argued that an overall strategy is not desirable and that services should develop in response to local needs. This seems to have been the sentiment of the DHSS document of 1975, which states:

> '... the planning of psychiatric nursing services for the future still needs to relate nurse staffing to the total needs of the population rather than to one particular type of facility ... as the pattern of services changes, so it will be necessary to change the pattern of deployment of nursing staff within the district and it will be one of the responsiblities of local nursing management to decide how best to deploy staff between the different elements of the district services.'

This statement clearly defines the local nurse managers as being responsible for service provision. Mangen and Griffith (1982) maintain that service development must be debated at national level. The authors assert that the continued expansion of community psychiatric nursing services must be assessed within psychiatric nursing as a whole and be closely related to manpower planning in mental health care. This cannot take place without statistical information.

In reviewing the state of development of community psychiatric nursing services, it is clear that they have developed differently and locally. Two questions emerge. First, do the services being developed meet local needs, and are service priorities set at local level? Second, are the assumptions involved in service development made explicit? These questions had a major effect on the present study and directed the enquiry to an evaluation of local community psychiatric nursing services. This evaluation was from the viewpoint of the family, on the one hand, and the assumptions of the community psychiatric nurses, on the other.

3 | The study

APPLICATION OF THE LITERATURE REVIEW

The aims and objectives of the present study have already been detailed in chapter 1. Before going on to detail the work, a summary will be made of the literature review, in order to refocus the attention of the reader on the concern of this study.

The literature review has shown that there are very few 'outcome' studies of community psychiatric nursing, and that those that have been done have been on specific diagnostic groups of patients. The review also revealed that the 'process' of community psychiatric nursing has escaped intensive study by previous researchers.

The way in which community psychiatric nurses actually work is worthy of close scrutiny, particularly because little is known about the nature of the work in practice. Knowledge about community psychiatric nursing is based on a quantitative data-base and is limited to the *theory* of how community psychiatric nurses work. The work of community psychiatric nursing has not previously been explored, nor examined, in order to ascertain whether or not nurses put the 'theory into practice'. It was considered to be a valuable exercise to examine the work more closely and find out how the nurses view it. This would then provide a sound foundation for the future development of community psychiatric nursing services; current development, as the review has shown, is haphazard and uneven.

The literature also suggested that the work of community psychiatric nursing is stated in vague and imprecise terms; this mirrors the ambiguity and confusion surrounding definitions of 'community care' at the policy-making level. It was, therefore, felt to be worth investigating one community psychiatric nursing service to discover from the nurses in the practice situation whether they worked with a common purpose, and to explore whether the goals, assumptions and values of community psychiatric nurses could be discerned with clarity.

Exploration of the term 'community care' showed that its meaning was varied and confusing. Review of the concept showed that resources 'in' the community are limited and that there is a dual emphasis in current government policy: to promote care 'for' the community (i.e. to increase the caring potential of the community) and to avoid institutional care (and rather encourage care 'by' the family). The literature further suggested that community psychiatric nurses theoretically have a role to play with the families of patients who are mentally ill and cared for at home. In particular, the review showed that nurses would be able to 'support the carers' by relieving 'burden', reducing expressed emotion and providing 'continuity of care'.

The above comments on the effect of policy on informal carers, combined with the lack of 'outcome' studies in community psychiatric nursing, led to the decision to produce an 'outcome' measure of community psychiatric nursing by examining the carers' view of the helpfulness of community psychiatric nursing contact. Furthermore, it was hoped to look at the 'fit' between the goals expressed by the nurses and those perceived by the carers.

The following study, therefore, emerged, which aimed to evaluate community psychiatric nursing firstly at the level of individual practice, to provide qualitative information about the 'process' of community psychiatric nursing, both generally and more specifically in relation to carers nursing mentally-ill patients at home. Secondly, this study focused on 'outcome' by providing feedback from the carers about their view of community psychiatric nursing work and about problem relief in relation to community psychiatric nursing intervention.

Review of the growth of community psychiatric nursing as a speciality showed that the development of community psychiatric nursing services is local in nature. For this reason, it seems logical to study community psychiatric nursing at a local level. The work of two different community psychiatric nursing services is described and compared in order to establish the way in which community psychiatric nurses work. The carers' views of these community psychiatric nursing services and of nursing helpfulness were also obtained.

THE LOCAL CONTEXT OF THE STUDY

In the following section, a description is given of the two hospitals and community psychiatric nursing services where the study took place. A summary of these details can be found in tables 1 and 2 below.

The setting of the study: East and West Hospitals

The hospitals included in the study remain anonymous. This decision was the researcher's, and was based on the fact that a central feature of the study was the analysis of the practice of individual community psychiatric nurses. Obscuring the names of the hospitals serves to protect the individual community psychiatric nurses who may otherwise have been identifiable. To protect the identity of the few male community psychiatric nurses in the study, the convention of referring to all the individual community psychiatric nurses as 'he' is adopted.

The parent hospitals

The term 'parent' is used here to describe the hospital which employed the community psychiatric nurses; in practice the nurses' work would not necessarily entail daily contact with the hospital. Each of the parent hospitals, as they existed at the time of the fieldwork for the study (see figure 2 below), is described separately below in the text. Table 1 summarises the details of these descriptions.

Table 1 Summary of the descriptions of the parent hospitals in the data collection sites

East Hospital	West Hospital
	Rural setting
	Unified administrative structure
	Training area for nurses, OTs, social workers and psychologists
	Eclectic use of models
Psychogeriatric beds	
Two thirds of total	One third of total
Hospital size: smaller	Larger
Medical cover	
By trainees and trained psychiatrists; by catchment area	Trained psychiatrists; by sectorisation
Community facilities	
Full range of services offered	More limited resources
Variety of day care services	No community day care
A number of group homes	No group home

NB: Similarities between the two services are detailed in the centre of the table. Differences appear in columns under the respective hospital.

East Hospital   East Hospital was situated in a rural setting in a mining area and covered a population of approximately 100 000. A small Victorian-built psychiatric hospital, it had almost 300 beds and provided the full range of psychiatric services; two-thirds of the inpatient beds were for psychogeriatric patients, but there were an acute admission unit and three rehabilitation wards. The hospital functioned as three units – psychogeriatric, rehabilitation and acute – and each had a consultant psychiatrist and a nursing officer. Within these units, each ward functioned as a clinical team; nurses provided the 24-hour care, but there was social worker, clinical psychologist and occupational therapist/occupational therapy helper input, which allowed the wards to believe they worked as multi-disciplinary teams.

In most areas, clinical methods of treatment were eclectic, but the 'medical model' approach to care predominated. In this, patients were seen in terms of medical diagnosis and the activities of the nurses were related to 'symptoms' – gathering information about symptoms to provide a diagnosis or to reduce the experience or effect of symptoms, by, for example, treatment, whether this was medication-giving, psychological or social. Combined with its clinical functions, the hospital was a training area for students and trainees in a variety of disciplines: nursing, psychiatry, general medicine, clinical psychology and social work.

The extramural facilities offered by the parent hospital were varied. A day centre and a supervised group home were situated in the hospital grounds; these provided the opportunity for patients to be discharged gradually from the hospital setting. Additionally, there was a range of day-care facilities and group homes available for use by patients, either pre- or post-hospitalisation. A degree of unanimity was maintained within the parent hospital through unified administrative structures and professional groups, and through periodic movements of staff in training.

West Hospital   West Hospital was a small, Victorian-built psychiatric hospital which served the psychiatric needs of approximately 300 000 people. The surrounding mining area was mainly rural but there were small pockets of population. Bigger than East Hospital, it had almost 650 beds and more than double the number of wards, one third of which were for psychogeriatric patients. Three nursing officers were responsible for three functional units in the hospital: acute, psychogeriatric and rehabilitation. Additionally there were a night-duty and a 'community' nursing officer.

In some respects the hospital offered a limited psychiatric service: patients were discharged straight into the community as there were no hostels or group homes to provide a graded discharge, and there were no day centres situated near the hospital. There was a recently-built day hospital attached to the parent hospital, which provided separate day care for 25 psychogeriatric and acutely-ill patients. Clincially, the work was similar to that of East Hospital, and the medical model approach to care predominated.

The hospital was not an accredited training hospital for medical, psychiatric or general practice students, but all other disciplines had training placements in West Hospital. Medical cover, by trained psychiatrists responsible to the consultant in charge, was organised on the basis of 'sectorisation', where each doctor had responsibility for a defined geographical area.

The community psychiatric nursing services
In the following text, the community psychiatric nursing services of the two parent hospitals are described in detail. The differences and similarities of the two services are summarised in table 2.

Table 2 Summary of the descriptions of the community psychiatric nursing services in the two data collection sites

East Hospital	West Hospital
	Developed from aftercare services
	Services began in 1960s
	Organised centrally, by CPN/NO, who also has hospital responsibilities
	Nurses work 9–5pm
	One trained CPN
	One nurse undergoing training
Catchment-wide service	Sectorised service
Weekend cover provided	No weekend service
Consultant referral system	Open referral system, active GP liaison
The CPNs	
Total number: 8	Total number: 10
Grades: assorted (CNs, SNs, ENs)	Grades: all CNs
Less experienced	More experienced
A hospital-based team	
Plus three day centre bases	Plus three general hospital centre bases
No planned, regular contact with hospital wards	
A more static day-care service	Domiciliary/community work
Specialist function/work-load	Generic function/work-load
CPNs have shared clients	CPNs have personal clients

NB. Similarities between the two services are detailed in the centre of the table. Differences appear in columns under the respective hospital.

East Hospital The eight community psychiatric nurses, of various grades (see below), had worked in the community team at the hospital for between two and six years. The service began as a follow-up service in the mid-1960s. Costs were initially met from the hospital budget; thus, the development was at the expense of hospital staffing. By the time of the study, all but three of the community posts had been transferred to a different budget.

Only one of the charge nurses was specifically trained for work as a 'community psychiatric nurse'. Another of the charge nurses was seconded, part-time, on a community psychiatric nursing course for the duration of the study. The experience of individuals in psychiatric nursing before appointment to the community team ranged from two to fifteen years. Two nurses were also general nurse trained. The community psychiatric nurses, in addition to formal training, received in-service training and opportunities to attend study days and conferences.

There was a nursing officer in charge of the community psychiatric nursing service in East Hospital, who had overall responsibility for co-ordinating and monitoring the service. This was a joint appointment, in that, although he had an active clinical role in the community psychiatric nursing team, he also had a service commitment to the parent hospital. This involved providing hospital senior nurse cover, on a rota basis, for early mornings, evenings and weekends.

The remaining nursing component of the community psychiatric nursing service operated from two different bases and exhibited a certain amount of specialisation of function. There was the hospital-based team which comprised two charge nurses and an enrolled nurse. Each had designated responsibility for specific patient groups: one charge nurse worked with the psychogeriatric patients and the other with the acutely ill, while the enrolled nurse worked predominantly with 'chronic' patients and was responsible for the supervision of the four group homes and for the running of an injection clinic. The nature of the work of these nurses was the provision of a home-visiting service.

There were also 'day centre' based community psychiatric nurses, who worked from three satellite day centres; these staff consisted of two charge nurses, one staff nurse and one enrolled nurse. Each of these day centres was described as having responsibility for provision of care to a distinct 'type' of patient and each was organised differently.

Two part-time day centres, for ambulant confused elderly, were run by the staff nurse (with the support of an occupational therapy helper). These were in local community centres, whose layout and toilet facilities were considered inadequate for the purpose. The day centres provided diversional activities for the elderly; this, combined with home-visiting, was considered to provide a respite service for carers.

A day unit for 'chronic patients', run by one of the charge nurses with support from an occupational helper, provided therapeutic programmes aimed at rehabilitation, the provision of 'working, domestic recreational and social pursuits' and a home-visiting service. A third day centre, organised by an enrolled nurse and a charge nurse (with social work support), was developed for 'personality disordered' patients as an alternative to the traditional treatment offered by the hospital setting. The expressed aim of the day centre was 'to prevent hospitalisation . . . bring psychiatry into the context of the family and community, in the hope of diminishing the stigma attached to mental illness'. This was accomplished by means of group therapy on a day-care basis and home-visiting by the community psychiatric nurses. A weekly injection clinic was also held at this centre.

Each community psychiatric nurse provided a 9a.m.–5p.m. service. An 'on-call' service (which the nurses described as a 'crisis intervention service', see p.29), operated on a 24-hour basis, seven days a week. Emergency requests (from GPs or the parent psychiatric hospital) for psychiatric assessment at the weekend were dealt with by joint visits of the 'on-call' nurse and the duty psychiatrist. The majority of referrals to the community psychiatric nurses were via consultant psychiatrists from the parent hospital. Direct GP referral of ex-patients was occasionally accepted. Two of the charge nurses attended the consultant's outpatient clinics, from where referrals were received.

The above quotations are from a printed pamphlet describing one of the day centres. The therapeutic atmosphere created there, was 'deliberately informal'; that of the hospital base and remaining day centres was similarly relaxed, with business and patient interactions conducted in a joking and flippant manner.

West Hospital There were 10 community psychiatric nurses in the second study area. All of these were employed at charge nurse grade and had worked in the community team at the hospital for two to 12 years. This service had started as an after-care service, almost 15 years previously. All the 'community posts' were separately funded.

One of the charge nurses was specifically trained for work as a 'community psychiatric nurse', and for the duration of the study period one of the charge nurses was seconded on a full-time community psychiatric nursing course. The experience of individuals in psychiatric nursing before appointment to the community team ranged from 12 to 30 years; therefore, this group was an older and more experienced group than that in East Hospital. In addition to the psychiatric training, two of the nurses were dual-trained, one as a general nurse and the second having completed a post-basic training in family therapy. As in East Hospital, the community psychiatric nurses received in-service training and opportunities to update knowledge by attendance at study days and conferences in addition to formal training.

The community psychiatric nursing service was managed and organised by a nursing officer who occasionally 'covered' the parent hospital; the nursing officer was responsible for the organisation and management of all the community psychiatric nurses whose offices were in hospitals separate from the parent psychiatric hospital. At the time of the study, the nursing officer's post was vacant due to promotion of the previous post-holder.

From the outset, it was apparent that this service offered a different perspective from that in East Hospital, where the service was more static and day care based (see chapter 4). In West Hospital, all the community psychiatric nurses actively liaised with the GPs and an open referral system operated. The service emphasised the 'generic' role of the community psychiatric nurses, although individual nurses' skills and preferences necessitated some specialism. At the request of GPs, the community psychiatric nurses provided 'home assessments' and arranged for holiday admissions of patients suffering from dementia to the parent hospital; the community psychiatric nurses did not retain these patients on their case-loads nor did they provide regular visits.

The community psychiatric nurses in West Hospital worked from four different bases: the parent psychiatric hospital and three satellite general hospitals. The catchment area of West Hospital was divided into north and south. Each area was covered by community psychiatric nurses operating from two bases, each of these catering for a specific geographical area.

One of the bases in the southern region was the parent hospital, and three of the community psychiatric nurses worked from there. One of these was on the community psychiatric nursing course; details of his work are not included in this study. The remaining two were partly attached to local GP practices, from whom direct referrals were received. Much of the work was with anxiety- and stress-related disorders, and both nurses shared the running and organisation of a depot clinic. Another community psychiatric nurse worked in the southern region; he worked mostly with consultant referrals doing a range of activities including anxiety management, group work and provision of medication.

The remaining community psychiatric nurses served the northern catchment area of the hospital and worked from two different bases. The first base was an office in the administrative suite of a small, modern district general hospital; here, two community psychiatric nurses worked. Both of the charge nurses worked with chronic schizophrenic patients and ran a social support group: one organised the depot clinics and organised social skills groups, while the other concentrated on group work for people with anxiety management problems and ran (with a trained addiction counsellor from the local social services) a self-help group for drug-dependent people. In addition to the work mentioned, these nurses provided a home-visiting and assessment service. The charge nurses received referrals from the consultant psychiatrists at the parent hospital and from the psychiatrists based at the district general hospital which had two psychiatric wards.

The second base was also in a small general hospital; here, four community psychiatric nurses shared the same base as the district nurses. There was no psychiatric ward in this hospital.

In response to the lack of day centres in the region, one of these community psychiatric nurses had been appointed to provide a 'mobile day care service' similar to that described by Shires (1977). There were plans to expand this service to one with a team approach, but, at the time of the study, the community psychiatric nurse alone provided day care, on a sessional basis, in various venues scattered throughout the region. The care offered was related to the community psychiatric nurse's skills, and was specifically aimed at preventing hospital admission of people who 'often had disordered lives and were in need of support over crises'. This community psychiatric nurse organised 'stress control skills groups'; 'a prescribed drug abusers group', aimed at helping to stop the abuse of anxiolytic medicines; 'analytical groups' using transactional analysis; and 'social treatment groups' aimed at helping 'young adults to cope with relationship difficulties and develop appropriate adaptive behaviour'. This nurse was involved in marital therapy with couples, and saw clients on an individual basis. Referrals were from local GPs and from one psychiatrist at the parent hospital.

Of the remaining three nurses at the second base, two received referrals of ex-patients from the parent hospital consultant and organised the injection clinic, support groups, and a home-visiting and assessment service. The third nurse received mostly GP referrals and was actively involved in 'helping people grow and develop out of the sick role', using individual case-work approaches, joint work with families and couples and group therapy techniques.

The individual community psychiatric nurses provided a 9a.m.–5p.m. service and, in contrast to East Hospital, there was no 'on-call' or crisis intervention service.

THE RESEARCH PLAN

The research plan for the study comprised three successive phases. During the first phase, pilot work took place in relation to the two chosen methods used in the study (see below). The first phase was followed by two main data collection phases, one in East Hospital, the other in West Hospital. To assist the reader in following the various phases, they are set out in the form of a diagram (figure 2) which also details when each phase took place and its duration.

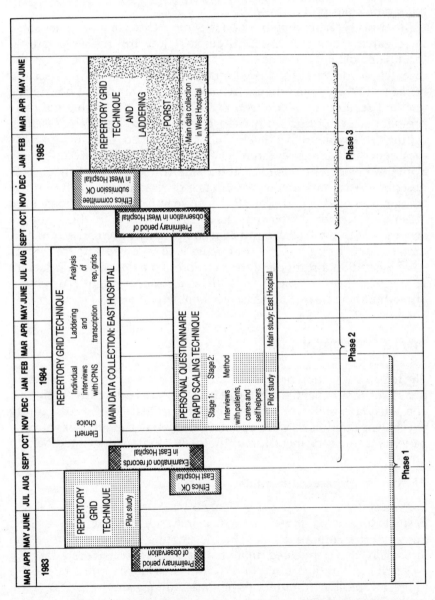

Figure 2 Diagram showing phases of data collection during the present study

Each main data collection phase was preceded by a preliminary period of observation, spent attached to the community psychiatric nurses being studied, when I was able to familiarise myself with the work and geographical area covered by the community psychiatric nurses. This also enabled me to form relaxed relationships with the community psychiatric nurses, nursing management in the hospital and other professionals in contact with the community psychiatric nurses, and to organise the practicalities of implementation of the main data collection phases.

Altschul (1972a) commented on the importance of a pre-pilot stage in research studies in order to get to know the research setting, formulate plans and make decisions about implementing the research, a point also made by Lofland and Lofland (1984). Rossi and Williams (1972) commented, 'Instance after instance can be cited of strained relationships between evaluators and the evaluated'. The pre-pilot stages of this study helped me to get to know the research settings and avoided the development of 'strained relationships'. My experience of 'doing research' was more akin to that described by Spradley (1980) who talked of 'the insider/outsider experience'. This describes the simultaneous experience of feeling part of the setting being researched yet, at other times, of feeling like an outsider. Lack of strained relationships may have been related to the pre-pilot activities or to my background as a community psychiatric nurse. A drawback of 'being known' and being well received was that I may have missed important data; furthermore, I may have been reluctant to question the nurses as stringently as a stranger might. The choice of method may have compensated somewhat for this.

THE MAIN STUDY

The following section provides details of the two main data collection phases of the present study, which took place consecutively in East and West Hospitals. Information about the choice of the community psychiatric nursing services and the selection of the subjects (nurses, patients, carers) for inclusion in the main study is presented below.

The choice of parent hospitals

East Hospital
East Hospital was chosen as a research site because the nursing officer of the community psychiatric nursing team approached me informally and requested that this service be considered for any research I was undertaking. In the absence of any criteria on which to judge a 'typical' community psychiatric nursing service (p.23), there seemed no reason to refuse the nursing officer's request.

The criterion of 'newness' is used to determine research sites. Struening and Guttentag (1975) have noted, 'The old established program is rarely a candidate for research. It is the new and innovative program that is put on trial while the hardy perennials go on, thro' sheer weight of tradition, whether or not they are accomplishing their goals'. Bearing these comments in mind, it was decided to examine a community psychiatric nursing service of the 'hardy perennial' type; the long-standing and stable nature of the service based at East Hospital fulfilled this specification and the service was, therefore, chosen.

West Hospital

The study was extended to a second site, environmentally similar to the first, the intention being to see how far the findings in East Hospital were borne out and which, if any, were weakened. Despite the initial similarities of the hospitals and the community psychiatric nursing services, closer examination revealed that there were also marked differences (see above).

Gaining access

East Hospital

Access to community psychiatric nurses The existing health board policy regarding 'access' for nursing research in East Hospital required a 'top down' approach, via the nursing hierarchy. Permission was, accordingly, granted to approach staff in East Hospital and, as already stated, the nursing officer was pleased to be involved. The participation of the community psychiatric nurses was voluntary, but it is doubtful that the individual nurses felt entirely free to opt out of a project sanctioned by senior staff. The friendly, open and welcoming manner of the community psychiatric nurses, and the fact that they co-operated in the study, which made considerable demands on their time, patience and energy, suggested that any doubts that existed about the research or myself had been shelved.

Access to patients and carers During the preliminary period of observation, the study was discussed with senior medical and nursing staff. As the research was non-intrusive, it was at first considered unnecessary to take the proposed research to the ethics committee. Before final permission was granted to do the research, the study was discussed at the Hospital Multi-disciplinary Management Group; they considered that the involvement of patients warranted scrutiny of the study by the local ethics committee. Written application for approval by the ethics committee was sought and given, but not without delay (see figure 2).

Contact names and addresses of patients and their respective carers were needed for both the pilot and the main study. The community psychiatric nursing and medical staff approved the final list of names to ensure that there were no clinical reasons which may have militated against me approaching any individual; no name was removed from the initial list.

Patients were specifically asked if they were willing to talk to me about the community psychiatric nursing service and also to complete a questionnaire. No formal consent form was signed. No advance warning was given of the research or my visit (see p.109). With the exception of carers of demented patients, permission of individual patients was sought prior to a carer being approached.

West Hospital

Access to community psychiatric nurses   As in East Hospital a 'top down approach' was made, via the nursing hierarchy, to gain permission to do the research with the community psychiatric nurses in West Hospital. Accordingly, the reservations about the 'voluntary' participation of the nurses, mentioned above, are relevant here. This did not seem to produce an adverse reaction: the community psychiatric nurses were, in fact, extremely obliging and were interested in and welcoming of the research activities.

Access to patients and carers   An approach to the ethics committee was mandatory in the second area of data collection and involved appearing in person to 'justify the study'. Two main outcomes resulted from this, both of which were related to safeguarding access to the patients' records. First, medical staff (the consultant in charge) had to give written agreement to individual patients entering the study (see appendix I); this form was designed by myself. Second, patients had to sign a consent form (see appendix II). Use of a form designed specifically for this study was not allowed; the form provided was for the patients' use, and more appropriate for medical trials.

A lengthy debate about the deliberations of the ethics committee is inappropriate here, but it should be noted that the preoccupation of the committee was concern for the patient. Although, by implication, information about the carer was also protected, carer consent was neither discussed nor specifically requested. The signing of a consent form was considered unnecessary by the researcher and may have biased the responses. The respondents accepted the consent procedure as a matter of course.

Approach to the patients and carers was as for East Hospital; before doing the research questionnaire, all respondents were asked to complete the consent form which was explained as a requirement of the committee which had allowed me to do this study.

Selection of the community psychiatric nurses

East Hospital
During the preliminary period of observation in East Hospital, I had to decide which nurses should be involved in the study. I was confronted with the issue of who should be defined as 'a community psychiatric nurse'. Perhaps surprisingly, members of the same 'community psychiatric nursing team' had differing views on whether they considered themselves to be community psychiatric nurses. Some said they were not 'community psychiatric nurses' but saw themselves, rather, as 'hospital psychiatric nurses working in the community'. This may have been an artefact of the research – the nurses becoming anxious at being the subjects of research and fearful that they were being judged against criteria of community psychiatric nursing practice for which they were not specifically trained. The uncertainty about the use of the term 'community psychiatric nurse' referred to in the literature is also relevant to the practitioners.

The reaction against being called a 'community psychiatric nurse' was exclusively limited to those nurses who worked from a day centre base. I considered excluding the day-centre nurses but decided not to do this, as the nursing officer saw these nurses to be 'community psychiatric nurses' and different from the hospital-based psychiatric nurses. So, all eight nurses in the 'East' team took part in the research.

West Hospital
The difficulties of definition, apparent for the nurses based in East Hospital, were not evident in West Hospital. All the nurses in the 'community psychiatric nursing team' considered themselves to be 'community psychiatric nurses'; none of the community psychiatric nurses of West Hospital were involved in day-centre work. Four of West Hospital's community psychiatric nurses were chosen, one community psychiatric nurse per geographical base. Of a total of 10 community psychiatric nurses, three were excluded from the study (one was away on a course, a second was about to go on maternity leave and a third was due to retire); of the seven remaining, two were chosen by process of elimination, two randomly.

Selection of the patients

East Hospital

Record keeping The community psychiatric nurses kept two kinds of records relating to patient contact. First, they filled in 'statistical returns', which were hospital forms requiring quantitative details for administrative purposes; these recorded the 'actual' attendances of patients at the day centres. The traditional format of the nursing 'Kardex' (a loose-leaf holder containing a running record of details of the nursing contact which took place with patients) was also used. This, in comparison, included *any* contact which the community psychiatric nurses had had, which was *to do with* the patient. This included direct contact at a day centre, home visit, or outpatient appointment, and also included more indirect contacts, e.g. telephone calls by or about the patient, and contact with family, GP or carers. Entries were also made if a patient had missed an appointment.

Comparison of the statistical returns with Kardex entries did not necessarily tally; there were more recorded attendances in the statistical returns. This suggests, therefore, that not all attendances at the day centre were recorded in the nursing Kardexes. From cursory examination of the Kardexes (by scanning the content of the entries), entries tended to be made if the community psychiatric nurses were actively engaged in problem resolution; patients who had been on the books for a long time had fewer entries than 'newer' patients.

Contrary to my expectation, each community psychiatric nurse did not have his own case-load; instead, there was a 'communal' case-load. Different nurses, therefore, visited the same patient (on different occasions), although it was noted that a few patients were visited by one community psychiatric nurse if consistency of input was required. This finding had implications for the choice of patients to be included in the main study. Based on the assumption that all the patients knew each psychiatric nurse, random selection of patients would produce feedback about all the community psychiatric nurses. However, conversation with individual community psychiatric nurses suggested that each did, in practice, seem to have his own patients, and different community psychiatric nurses specialised in certain types of work. The nursing Kardexes were, therefore, examined to find out if the case-load was truly 'common'.

Examination of the nursing records   To establish a sampling frame, the signed entries in the nursing Kardexes were examined by the researcher; this took one month. This examination showed that more than half of the patients were in contact with one community psychiatric nurse, suggesting that the nurses did not have a common pool of patients. Patients, however, who attended the day centres had contact with three or more nurses. It was decided, therefore, that the sample of patients would be related to contact with individual community psychiatric nurses. The entries for each patient visited or in contact with more than one community psychiatric nurse were examined more closely, and the nurse who had written *most* Kardex entries (over a six-month period) was identified and considered to be the 'key worker'. (The nursing officer had few patients for whom he could be described as the key worker; he had hospital and weekend administrative work, leaving limited time for direct patient care. The nurse seconded to the community psychiatric nursing course, working on a reduced case-load, also had fewer patients with whom to be identified as the key worker.)

Visiting frequency by the community psychiatric nurses Another factor noted during examination of the nursing Kardexes was the wide range of 'frequencies' of contact with patients. This, of course, was not a totally unexpected finding, for two reasons: first, on a clinical level, varying patients' needs dictate varied community psychiatric nursing input; second, Sladden (1979) commented that the community psychiatric nurses in her study were reluctant to discharge patients from the books. The fact that some patients on the records were not seen at all for six months suggested that this latter situation may also have been the case in East Hospital.

The patient sample To examine this aspect of the 'process' of community psychiatric nursing, the subjects for inclusion in the main study were chosen on the basis of frequency of visits. This decision was influenced by the work of Bloch (1975), who suggested that examination of the 'process' of nursing activity should be linked with examination of 'outcome'. It was hoped that frequency of visits of the community psychiatric nurses ('process') in the present study could be linked with the outcome of the service (evaluation by the carers).

Another major factor which affected the choice of sample was that previous evaluative research into the work of the community psychiatric nurse has tended to focus on specialist patient populations, defined by diagnosis (see p.41). This research intended to focus on the whole range of patients visited by community psychiatric nurses. From personal experience in clinical work, frequency of visiting is related to the condition of the patient (the more acutely disturbed patients tend to be visited more frequently) and what the nurse is doing during the visit (intensive family work may demand more frequent visits than routine assessments). Based on this rationale, it was assumed that a sample which covered patients with a range of frequency of visits would provide a sample of patients with varied conditions, illnesses, and needs, and would also reflect a range of inputs and therapies on the part of the community psychiatric nurses.

Seven patients were chosen for each community psychiatric nurse. The patients were listed in order of frequency of visits: the most and least frequently visited patients were selected, plus five others evenly spaced throughout the remaining list. This sample reflects each nurse's input, and could broadly be described as that of a stratified sample based on frequency of visiting by the community psychiatric nurses (as recorded in the nursing Kardexes).

West Hospital

As in East Hospital, the community psychiatric nurses completed statistical returns and patient contacts were recorded in a nursing Kardex. Examination of the records to work out a 'key worker' was unnecessary in West Hospital because each community psychiatric nurse had a personal case-load. To facilitate comparison of findings, selection of patients here was as that described above, based on examination of the individual nursing Kardexes and frequency of visiting.

Selection of carers in East and West Hospitals

For each patient chosen for the main study, the name and address of the next of kin, as recorded in the nursing Kardex, was noted. Using the guidelines suggested by Platt et al (1980), the patient (unless he was demented) was asked to identify the carer with whom he was most in contact; this usually coincided with the next of kin given in the Kardex, the exceptions being for couples who were separated.

THE METHODS

This final section of chapter 3 focuses on the two methods used in the present study. An overview of each method is provided and the rationale given for these choices; the advantages of each are summarised and the techniques of data analysis are presented. Both methods were the subject of pilot studies which are also detailed.

Methodology

Various methods were explored prior to the decision to use those described below. In attempting to think back to the other methods considered and the reasons for their rejection, the comments of Kratz (1974) became particularly relevant. This author stated:

> 'Literature of particular relevance to one's chosen field is scarce; because of this, one casts one's net wide, in an effort to find something, anything which might be useful in throwing light on the vast emptiness by which one is surrounded. In the end, one's reading becomes so wide as to become almost unconnected with one's point of departure. Some of it is forgotten, the relevance of much, which at the time seemed central to the theme under investigation, becomes dimmed. Other material grows from relative insignificance to become the focal point of one's thinking. Yet somehow all items, whether only dimly remembered, superceded by

events, or growing in importance, have contributed to one's thinking and to the finished work.'

These comments reveal that doing research is a 'process' and that it is an almost impossible task to recollect the details of the process which shaped any piece of research. This study is no exception, and the shortfalls in the recall and reporting of this process must be acknowledged. What have been remembered are the various methodological landmarks which signposted the direction and which were responsible for the study taking its present form. These are summarised below. The retrospective nature of this summary gives the path a more organised appearance than that actually experienced, and does not give credit to the influence of the researcher's informal contact with peers and fellow students which also affected the emergent study. Other factors like time, skill and labour availability also had a bearing on the study methodology.

At the outset, it was envisaged that the way in which the nurses worked and the effect that this had on carers could be examined simultaneously. Observational methods which had been predominantly used in the past to study the work of psychiatric nurses (Oppenheim and Eeman, 1955; John, 1961; Altschul, 1972b; Towell, 1975; Cormack, 1976) were reviewed and considered for use in the present study. The review showed that an observational approach to psychiatric nursing had failed to identify crucial components of the work, which were not amenable to direct observation. Some researchers, notably McIlwaine (1980), supplemented direct observation by using a radio microphone to record patient/nurse interactions. Nevertheless, observational techniques examine behaviour as it occurs and are, therefore, less effective in explaining behaviour.

This study was conceived with the aims of finding out the goals, assumptions and values of the community psychiatric nurses and of evaluating nurses' performance in the light of these goals; the observational method did not seem to offer opportunity to explore these aspects of the nurses' work. Examination of what the nurses did and said to carers in the domiciliary setting would also provide little information on the 'outcome' of any interaction. Previous attempts at using 'observation' of patients and clients in the home situation (documented by Sladden, 1979) were unsuccessful, because clients tried to engage the 'observer' in the interaction.

The survey method, sometimes called 'the poor man's experiment' (Oppenheim, 1983), was then considered, but was rejected on the grounds that this aimed at gathering census-like data and was essentially a fact-finding exercise. It seemed, initially at least, that previous studies had provided enumerative data, both on the work of community psychiatric nursing (Community Psychiatric Nurses Association, 1985b) and on the experience of carers of the mentally ill (see p.49), and that using this approach in the present study would add little to current knowledge.

Consideration then moved towards examination of less descriptive and more analytical methods using more tightly controlled designs. These initially seemed attractive with regard to evaluating community psychiatric nursing services (see Paykel and Griffith, 1983; Brooker, 1984b) because they offered the opportunity to look at the relations between variables and allowed for inferences and predictions to be made. Somehow, this move from looking at survey design to experimental methods guided me into focusing on the literature which compared taking a qualitative with a quantitative approach.

This, in turn, resulted in the search for appropriate methods being directed towards 'grounded theory' (Glaser and Strauss, 1967) which has been focused on recently as a useful research method for nurses (Simms, 1981; Melia, 1981; Powell, 1982; Field and Morse, 1985; Chenitz and Swanson, 1986). The reservation of using the grounded theory approach was that previous researchers had found that psychiatric nurses found it difficult to talk about their work (see Altschul, 1972b). Furthermore, I was somewhat daunted at the thought of using a method which would generate two large amounts of data (data from both nurses and carers) which required transcription and analysis.

Brown (1973) and Norris (1981) discussed the interpretation of qualitative data; the latter author referred to the 'repertory grid technique' and, hence, introduced me to the method which had a formative influence on the aims of the study. Repertory grid technique is a method which combines a qualitative and quantitative approach, and it seemed particularly attractive for this reason. The method also seemed to provide the structure which would direct the focus of the study and produce specific data on the goals of community psychiatric nursing work. At this stage, it was decided to take a separate approach to the 'outcome' of community psychiatric nursing.

The 'personal questionnaire rapid scaling technique' (PQRST) was chosen to explore 'outcome'; this method was recommended by researchers using repertory grid methods (e.g. Slater, 1978) as a structured means of obtaining individualised information. This seemed to be suitable in this study, interested in the carers' views, and the data obtained from the PQRST could be linked back to the nurses' data.

The two methods of data collection used in the study are described below. These are:

1.   Structured interviews were carried out with the community psychiatric nurses in an attempt to investigate the 'process' of

community psychiatric nursing and to explore the goals of the work as expressed by the nurses. These interviews were conducted in accordance with the format of the repertory grid technique (repgrid) outlined by Fransella and Bannister (1977) and the 'laddering' procedure detailed by Hinkle (1965).

2. The personal questionnaire rapid scaling technique (Mulhall, 1971) was used to examine 'outcome' in terms of the families' views of the helpfulness of community psychiatric nursing contact and of their views of the 'process' of community psychiatric nursing.

The repertory grid method

A step-by-step guide to the method of repertory grid technique was published by the researcher in the *Journal of Advanced Nursing* (Pollock, 1986a).

Repertory grid technique was developed as a methodological component of a theory of personality ('personal construct theory') proposed by the psychologist George Kelly (Kelly, 1955, 1963). Kelly believed that humans develop predictive hypotheses ('constructs') which are tested, modified or discarded in order to survive; he considered this to be an active process which influences and conditions how individuals see the world, and he believed that individuals build up a network of hypotheses (based on unique experiences) which is called a 'construct system'. Repertory grid technique offers the opportunity for an individual's 'construct system' to be elicited.

'Constructs' are treated as if they are bipolar dimensions of judgment in which a description always has an opposite: 'light' is nonsense without a sense of its opposite, which could be 'heavy' or 'dark'. This opposite may not always be the dictionary opposite but can be the semantic opposite which conveys individual meaning and understanding.

Repgrid has been used for management, educational and clinical purposes (see Pollock, 1986a). The merits of the technique for use in research are summarised below.

Advantages of repgrid technique

1. The individual focus of the technique provides an effective means of exploring an individual's perception.

2. The discipline involved in the application of the technique ensures that each interview is structured and that the conversation is controlled; the technique is constructive as it facilitates listening and the collection of pertinent material. (Compare this with the unstructured interview situation, when, at times, both interviewer

and interviewee are talking over each other, sentences may be finished off by the researcher and (mis)interpreted or suggestions may be made. The interviewer may not be so much 'listening' to what the other person is saying as preparing the next remark. The conversation can transgress from the topic at hand, to irrelevant issues.) Using repgrid, the interviewer is forced to keep quiet, and the rigour of the comparing and contrasting technique ensures that the interviewee gives uninterrupted elaborations.

3. Observer bias is reduced almost to zero and objectivity is maximised because the input from the interviewer is minimal (Stewart and Stewart, 1981).

4. The conversational format of the technique recommends its use (Smith and Kendall, 1963). According to Watson (1970), the format is not anxiety-provoking and the respondent is reassured that there is no right or wrong answer.

5. The method makes it difficult for the interviewee to interpret its aims and to introduce and maintain a systematic bias in the responses (Rowe, 1971).

6. The method systematically obtains qualitative data; the vocabulary of individual members of a group can then be examined or the descriptions analysed using a hermeneutic approach. This method has been used in pilot studies to help develop questionnaires which are meaningful to the respondents (Stewart and Stewart, 1981).

7. The results can also provide quantitative data which can complement the qualitative findings. These data can be analysed by principal component analysis (see below), the results of which can be presented visually and diagramatically, as well as mathematically (Slater, 1976).

Many of the advantages listed above, e.g. the lack of experimenter bias, the constructive use of time and the fact that the results are analysable, would be pertinent to any research study. Altschul (1972a, 1973) found that it was difficult to get the psychiatric nurses in her study to talk about the thoughts, feelings and perceptions behind their work. In the light of these findings, the individual focus of the repertory grid technique and its conversational format particularly recommended its use in the present study. It promised to be an ideal method which could help individual community psychiatric nurses to verbalise their perceptions of their work. Using 'typical psychiatric patients' as 'elements', the method was used to investigate the constructs which individual community psychiatric nurses produced.

The repertory grid technique

The technique has been described as a type of structured interview, the format of which enables the collection of individuals' descriptions ('constructs'). This elicitation of constructs is triggered by a sorting procedure ('triadic elicitation'), where the topics of interest ('elements') are written on cards. The technique involves three distinct stages: element choice, construct elicitation and grid construction. Each of these stages is explained below and each was piloted (see. p. 87 for details of and reasons for the pilot study of the repertory grid technique).

The laddering procedure

This is a procedure, described by Hinkle (1965), for eliciting increasingly superordinate constructs, that is, constructs of a higher order of abstraction than those initially elicited. It is a conversational technique developed from repertory grid, and is aimed at systematically obtaining information from an individual in order to explore the meaning of one given construct. McCall and Simmons (1969) have stated:

> 'In exploring for possible factors affecting some given variable, or for chains of causes and effects constituting a 'process' there appear to be two basic techniques ... the second is to ask people themselves to explain what happened and to give their reasons for acting as they did. The basic question is always why?'

In the laddering procedure, the interviewer repeatedly asks the question 'why?'. Wright (1970) demonstrated the clinical use of the technique by using it to explore the meaning of psychological symptoms, necessary, he argued, for behaviour change. The laddering procedure has had limited use in research application: Allsop (1980) and Hazelden (1981) used the procedure with teachers to explore the reasons for reading difficulties and truancy respectively.

According to Landfield (1971), the laddering procedure provides a tool for documenting conversation. This has been used by Allsop (1980) and Slater (1976). Hinkle's procedure has been called 'laddering up' from a construct. The laddering procedure is explained clearly and at length by Judkins (1976), Fransella and Bannister (1977), Stewart and Stewart (1981) and Wright (1970). Constructs can also be explored by 'laddering down', where the respondent is asked 'how' one side of the construct differs from the other (see Pollock, 1986a, for a summary of this procedure, and figure 3 for an example of the procedure of 'laddering up' as used in the present study). All the laddered conversations were audiotaped to allow for qualitative analysis of the interview data.

LP: What we are going to do today is talk through some of the things you told me about last time, and really it will be getting you to state the very obvious about your work. I want you to tell me in your own words about your work, what you do and why. I've taken the descriptions you gave last time and we'll go through them.

LP: Family support — not. Tell me how someone with family support differs from somebody who doesn't have it, just to give me an idea of what you are talking about.

F: If someone has family support you are getting a more objective picture of what is going on and you are getting somebody's other than the patient's views. If someone has family support, you'll find out quickly if there is anything going wrong, if there is adverse change in the situation. You may find the family tend to over-react and you are called to crises that are not really crises; in the crisis situation you are more likely to be able to keep them out of hospital if they have family support.

LP: OK, let's take these separately. Why do you like to get a more objective picture?

F: To get a broader picture. Most of the information you get is subjective. You get a broader view if you speak to the family — of what is going on and what you are dealing with.

LP: Why do you want to do that?

F: Because we are not treating an illness, we are treating an individual, and the only way to get to know them as a complete person is to get to know them.

LP: You want to get to know them as a complete person — why?

F: To provide a better standard of care, of comprehensive care.

LP: Why do you want to do that?

F: To give a good service. An illness and symptoms cannot be just treated, the person has got to be looked at as an individual in his or her entirety.

LP: Why would you want to hear if there was something going on?

F: Sometimes you do and sometimes you don't. We can maybe take action to prevent further crisis and prevent an admission or any further trauma to the patient.

LP: Why do that?

F: That is difficult. The nurse's job is not just treating people; we owe it to our patients to give as good a service as we can, and part of this is preventative medicine, primary care.

LP: Why is it useful for you to know if someone doesn't have support?

F: The CPN's information-gathering processes would be more difficult. We would have to look for other sources of information, like neighbours, which would have ethical implications. Or we may have to visit relatives who live a distance away.

LP: Why do that?

F: To get more information . . .

Figure 3   An example of the 'laddering up' procedure

Using the repertory grid technique, it was hoped that, from the data provided:

1. examination of the constructs would help to answer the following questions:
    i. What patient information do individual community psychiatric nurses perceive as relevant to their work?
    ii. Do individual community psychiatric nurses select different pieces of information?
2. analysis of elements and constructs would provide information on the questions:
    i. Do individual community psychiatric nurses have different perceptions in relation to patients?
    ii. Can individual community psychiatric nurses be identified as using specific models of care?

Using the laddering procedure would help to answer the following questions:

- Are individual community psychiatric nurses aiming for the same goals as regards treatment? What are these goals?
- How do the nurses view work with carers?
- Do the community psychiatric nurses, as a group, have a united philosophy of community care?
- How do the community psychiatric nurses make community psychiatric nursing work? Is there a pattern to community psychiatric nursing action?

The pilot study of the repertory grid technique

Ten community psychiatric nurses were approached and invited to complete repertory grids. These community psychiatric nurses were either members of the community psychiatric nursing professional organisation (The Community Psychiatric Nurses Association) or were colleagues and friends of the researcher (community psychiatric nurses not in contact with or involved with the community psychiatric nursing services in the main study). They lived in different areas of Scotland, some with specialised and others with generic case-loads, and they reflected a variety of experiences of community psychiatric nursing and lengths of service.

The reasons for a pilot study
A pilot study of repertory grid was necessary for the following reasons:

- to provide myself, as the researcher, with the opportunity to gain confidence and competence in the repertory grid technique and the laddering procedure;

- to provide the researcher with the opportunity to analyse some of the data obtained and gain an understanding of the computer programme and possible results;
- to gain practice in the use of tape-recording;
- to allow the frequency of sessions with community psychiatric nurses in the main study to be estimated and the programme schedule to be planned;
- to create the opportunity for methodological aspects of the interview situation to be revised prior to the main study.

The first three reasons centred around the needs of the researcher, whereas the remaining two had implications for the main studies.

The practicalities of the technique   As recommended by Allsop (1980), I needed to gain confidence in the practicalities of the technique. This involved discussion with other researchers who had experience with the method, followed by practice using the method with both the experienced researchers and with community psychiatric nurses.

The analysis   One of the grids from the pilot was analysed; this confirmed that quantitative analysis, using the 'Ingrid' software package (see below), was possible with the university's mainframe computer. Advice and help was also available to help with this.

Tape-recording   Pilot work with the tape-recorder allowed me to develop a check-list of activities which ensured that the tape-recording of interviews in the main study was uneventful (see appendix III), and showed that this, or my note-taking, did not upset any of the community psychiatric nurses.

Frequency of sessions   Information was needed about the demands of repertory grid technique, for example, the length of the procedure and toleration of the subjects, in order, firstly, to plan and organise the data collection in the main study and, secondly, to maintain the goodwill and co-operation of the community psychiatric nurses. The pilot work demonstrated that the time needed for the elicitation, laddering and rating was lengthy. As a result of this, each community psychiatric nurse, in the main study, was seen at least four times in order to:

1. acquire the names to be used with the elements (Each nurse was asked to choose someone who was typical of each 'patient type'; these names were then written in pencil on the back of index cards.);
2. elicit constructs;
3. ladder the constructs;
4. complete the rating grid.

Co-operation of interviewees A most important consideration addressed by the pilot study was the co-operation of the interviewees. Scott (1962) said that repertory grid technique is 'a relevant task for describing people ...', but he continues, 'It is cumbersome to administer and score and it is doubtful that a non-captive population of adults would submit willingly to it ...'. Taking account of these comments, it was necessary to use the technique with a group of community psychiatric nurses to find out whether they would be willing and able to do the technique (i.e. to comply with the sorting procedure, to produce constructs and to use rating scales to build up the grid itself). Mair (1966) emphasised the importance of giving a clear indication of the context within which grid data are to be collected, and pointed out that failure to do so would result in the respondent flicking from one context to another while constructing a grid. The pilot study was used to make sure that respondents understood the instructions and were able to carry out the procedures without confusion.

The community psychiatric nurses in the pilot study understood the instructions and enjoyed the technique. They were initially slow to sort the cards and provide constructs, and were anxious to know if they were carrying out the procedure correctly; in the introduction of the main study, subjects were told that there were no right or wrong answers, and they were given positive feedback during the procedure. By the sixth sort of the pilot, subjects found eliciting easier; repetition of constructs caused worry to some of the community psychiatric nurses. Shubachs (1975) commented that repeated constructs indicate those most relevant to the subjects; this was encouraged in the main study.

The format of the repertory grid technique

Element choice
Elements may be people, objects, activities or concepts, and they define the content of the structured interview. Elements should cover as wide a range of topics to be discussed as possible in order that the elicitation procedure is meaningful and succeeds in procuring a variety of constructs.

Stewart and Stewart (1981) outline 'rules for selecting elements'. In summary, elements should be: discrete; nouns or verbs; homogeneous (i.e. all people, all objects or all activities); and non-evaluative. They emphasise that:

> 'Elements really should be as precise as you can get them. An imprecise element, struck against another imprecise element or two to produce a construct, will not produce much clarity of contrast and therefore will not produce good clear constructs ... a rough scatter over the element area is acceptable.'

Elements also must be meaningful and relevant to the subjects being interviewed; according to Yorke (1978), this is a crucial methodological consideration. Stewart and Stewart (1981) comment about strategies open to the researcher for selecting the elements:

> '... you can supply elements, you can get them by free-response; or you can use eliciting questions. Either of the last two strategies puts you within reach of the interviewer-bias-free interviewing procedure that was one of our original goals. There is nothing stopping you mixing strategies, either, though you should be clear about why you do it; if you do mix strategies then *it is probably best to begin with any eliciting questions you want to use, then go on to free response, and finish with supplied elements, making sure you check that the interviewee knows them.*' (my italics)

In this study the elements were descriptions of patients. The choice of 'patient types' as elements fulfilled the first three 'rules' outlined. The pilot study (see figure 2) ensured that the elements were not evaluative and that they were relevant and meaningful to community psychiatric nurses. The format outlined in italics above was tested in the pilot run and used in the main study.

The choice of elements is related to the purpose of the interview; the purpose of this study was to look at the process of community psychiatric nursing. By using patient types as elements, it was hoped that constructs would emerge which gave an insight into the types of patient information that community psychiatric nurses found relevant to their work and that, from this, constructs could be explored to give details about the goals which community psychiatric nurses used in their work. One of the major aims of the pilot study was to find out whether use of the technique, as proposed, did in fact elicit the predicted data. This aim was successfully achieved.

In the pilot study, a meaningful list of elements (patient types) was achieved by asking the community psychiatric nurses to describe the work they did and with whom they did it (cf. the 'free-response' strategy detailed above by Stewart and Stewart, 1981). Between six and ten elements resulted and the list varied markedly between nurses. For example, some community psychiatric nurses used diagnostic groupings to describe their patients, while others used 'nursing diagnosis' (such as 'chronic', 'acute', 'able to help', 'unable to help', 'old', 'young'); the list was that relevant to the individual nurse. In the main study, to aid comparison between the community psychiatric nurses, 'supplied elements' were used for the triadic sorts. These arose from individual interviews and a 'free-response' session, but were checked for relevance with the whole group of community psychiatric nurses.

Construct elicitation
Six methods of eliciting constructs are presented in the literature. These methods are concisely presented in Fransella and Bannister

(1977). In the present study, the 'triadic' (also known as 'minimal context form') method of presenting elements was chosen to elicit the constructs, because it was the simplest and least time-consuming method available. This means that the elements are presented to the subject in sets of three; the respondent is asked to say how two are similar but are different from a third.

Several difficulties with the 'sorting procedure' emerged during the pilot study.

The first of these was the use of the word 'important'. The introduction given was, 'What I am interested in is the sort of information that you like to know about patients, that is useful for your work'. The question then asked was, 'I'd like you to tell me an important way in which two of these patients are alike and different from a third'. The word 'important' seemed to cause difficulties and the community psychiatric nurses asked, 'Important for what?' Interviews without the word 'important' caused less difficulty and did not lead to irrelevant descriptions being given of the patients, e.g. red hair–blonde hair. This format was, thus, used in the main study.

Secondly, in the pilot study, the community psychiatric nurses selected cards/elements at random. This caused repetition of some elements and omission of others. In the main study, pre-determined triadic sorts were presented to the community psychiatric nurses (see appendix IV). Kasper (1962) recommended systematic presentation of elements for research purposes when using the repertory grid; this also avoided tedious repetitions, and ensured that all the elements were sorted.

The last difficulty was in eliciting the grid's 'implicit pole'. The similarity description (the 'emergent pole', see figure 4 below) arises spontaneously from the sorting procedure; the 'implicit pole', in comparison, requires to be prompted. Epting et al (1971) evaluated the elicitation procedure needed to do this and recommended asking directly, 'What is the opposite?', or using the prompt 'as opposed to' to obtain the implicit pole. These alternatives were tested in the pilot run. Asking for an 'opposite' from the community psychiatric nurses tended to produce dictionary opposites. The 'as opposed to' prompt caused no difficulty and gave a more accurate insight into the descriptions used by the community psychiatric nurse. This was, therefore, used in the main study.

Grid construction

Constructs and elements can be integrated into a 'grid format' – elements are listed along the top, and constructs along the side, of a matrix (figure 4). The interviewee is then asked to allocate constructs to elements. Insertion of the information into a 'grid' format, with each element rated in terms of the construct, allows the primary data to be clearly presented and be available for discussion. The ability of

Figure 4 An example of a grid matrix, taken from the present study

Constructs (emergent pole — implicit pole):

1. Has responsibilities/family — Doesn't have
2. Is in sheltered housing — Is in sole charge
3. Gets on well with whom lives — Doesn't
4. House sparse — House comfy/clean
5. Works full-time — Doesn't
6. Unemployed — Works
7. Housewife — Not
8. I know well — Don't
9. Black — Looks clean
10. Fat and healthy — Gets emaciated
11. Can be touchy and aggressive — Not
12. Can be verbally aggressive — Not
13. Hysterical — Isn't
14. Chronic — Not

Element	1	2	3	4	5	6	7	8	9	10	11	12	13	14
15 Chronic, unlikely to change	6	4	1	1	6	1	1	1	1	1	4	1	1	6
14 Chronic, likely to change	4	4	4	1	6	1	1	1	1	1	3	3	6	1
13 New referrals	1	6	1	6	6	1	1	6	6	4	6	6	6	4
12 Outpatient	1	6	1	3	6	1	1	1	3	1	6	6	6	1
11 Physically ill	4	6	1	1	6	1	1	1	6	4	6	6	6	1
10 Inpatient contact	6	6	1	6	1	6	1	1	6	6	3	3	1	6
9 Mildly demented	6	2	1	6	6	1	6	1	3	1	6	6	6	1
8 Requested visits	1	6	1	6	6	1	1	3	6	4	6	6	6	1
7 GP referral	6	2	5	6	6	1	6	1	6	1	1	1	1	1
6 Depressive	6	3	4	6	6	1	3	3	3	6	6	6	6	1
5 At risk	6	6	1	3	6	1	1	1	6	1	6	6	6	1
4 Consultant referrals	6	5	6	5	1	6	6	3	6	1	1	1	1	4
3 Other medication	1	6	1	6	3	3	1	1	3	4	3	1	3	1
2 'Depot' patient	1	6	1	6	6	1	1	1	6	1	3	1	6	1
1 'Lithium' patient	2	6	1	6	6	1	1	1	6	4	6	6	6	6

implicit pole / CONSTRUCTS: *emergent pole*

Figure 4 (continued)

Element	#	Has epilepsy / Not	Demented / Not	Suicide risk / Not	Diagnosis decided / Not	Physical problems / Not	Manic depressive / Isn't	When well, personality nice / Neurotic	Out of hospital / In hospital	On I.M. / Isn't	Comes to no.7 / Doesn't	Needs bribing for bath / Doesn't	Helped by CPN / Isn't	Male / Female
Chronic, unlikely to change	15	6	6	6	1	6	6	1	1	1	6	1	1	6
Chronic, likely to change	14	6	6	6	1	6	6	1	1	1	1	6	1	1
New referrals	13	6	6	3	6	6	6	1	1	6	1	6	4	1
Outpatient	12	6	6	6	1	6	6	1	1	1	1	6	1	1
Physically ill	11	1	6	6	4	1	1	1	1	1	1	6	1	1
Inpatient contact	10	1	6	3	1	6	6	1	1	1	1	6	1	6
Mildly demented	9	6	1	6	1	6	6	1	1	6	6	6	1	6
Requested visits	8	6	4	6	4	1	6	1	1	6	1	6	1	1
GP referral	7	6	6	6	1	6	1	4	1	1	1	6	1	6
Depressive	6	6	6	6	6	1	6	1	1	6	6	6	4	1
At risk	5	6	6	6	1	6	6	1	1	1	1	6	1	1
Consultant referrals	4	6	6	1	1	6	6	3	1	1	1	6	1	1
Other medication	3	6	4	6	4	1	6	1	1	6	6	6	1	1
'Depot' patient	2	6	6	6	1	6	6	1	1	1	1	6	1	6
'Lithium' patient	1	6	6	6	6	6	1	1	1	6	1	6	1	1

CONSTRUCTS: *emergent pole* (bottom) / *implicit pole* (right) the technique to provide quantitative information which could be analysed using statistical packages (see below) seemed to be an advantage of the method.

The subjects are asked to rate the given elements according to a specified scale. Roth (1976) has argued that language categories are not simply bipolar; he believes that there is a relativistic quality in language descriptions, a dimensional quality which suggests a range of statements rather than a choice of two. The precise relation of our perception of people to language is not necessarily one of clear-cut dichotomies. This suggests that the use of a rating scale on a continuum would be more appropriate in handling choices than would mutually-exclusive, traditional, dichotomous choices (Kelly, 1955).

Using a rating scale, the subjects have the freedom to allocate the elements as they wish, and fine discriminations are possible. In the words of Bannister and Mair (1968), the use of a rating scale has the aim of:

'(giving) the subject as much freedom as possible to express his judgements and to throw the onus of formalising and quantifying onto post test statistical processing.'

The community psychiatric nurses were asked to compile a grid using a six-point rating scale.

The data analysis

The quantitative analysis
Computer analysis Traditionally, the most common method of analysis of data derived from the repertory grid method is quantitative analysis of the material in the grid matrix (see figure 4). There are numerous techniques open to facilitate analysis of the numerical data of the repertory grid. These consist of sophisticated and complicated methods of analysis by computer packages (see Pope and Keen, 1981; Thomas and Harri-Augstein, 1985, for an overview of the methods).

In the present study, the quantitative data derived from the grid matrixes was analysed using the 'Ingrid' programme (Slater, 1978). There were two reasons for this choice of analysis: firstly, in published studies, 'Ingrid' was the most popular method of analysis (Beail, 1985); and, secondly, this programme was available locally on the mainframe computer, using the 'Statistical Package for the Social Sciences' (Nie, 1975).

'Ingrid' analysis provided correlational data on constructs, scores indicating the relationships between elements, and a principal component analysis of the construct and element data. This analysis indicated the dispersal of constructs, and thus their relationships to each other, in terms of all the elements that were rated, and also showed the dispersal of the elements in terms of the constructs used to rate them. Slater (1978) states that the principal component analysis was developed:

'merely as a method for simplifying the records of a large number of correlated variables . . . by reducing them to a possible smaller number of independent measurements, ordered from largest to least according to the amount of variation they recorded.'

This analysis, although undertaken, did not illuminate the data: each nurse chose his own elements and constructs, so 'Ingrid' produced a number of personal profiles from which no trends emerged which seemed to have more general application. The 'Ingrid' analysis proved to be less helpful than expected and did not provide additional information to that gained from the 'laddering' interviews. Interpretation of the 'Ingrid' analysis goes beyond the bounds of the data and should, according to the seminal work on repertory grid technique, be negotiated with the respondent (see Pollock, 1986a); lack of time meant that this was not possible in this study.

The constructs gained from the repertory grid technique were also quantitatively examined using a method of categorisation, based on subject matter (see chapter 4) and 'content analysis' (Berelson, 1952).

Content analysis 'Content analysis' is 'a research technique for the objective, systematic, and quantitative description of the manifest content of communication' (Berelson, 1952). Berelson discusses content analysis in depth. He makes a distinction between 'what' is analysed and 'how', and outlines 17 uses of content analysis. One of these uses is, 'focusing on the substance of the content, where the primary concern is with the referents of symbols' (Berelson, 1952, p.27). This is relevant to the present study where content analysis was used to look at the differences and similarities between the community psychiatric nurses. Berelson states that:

'Content analysis can be no better than its system of categories . . . and should employ categories most meaningful for the particular problem at hand . . . relevant categories are limited only by the analysts' imagination in stating a problem.'

Nine 'types' of categories are suggested by Berelson. The first of these, related to subject matter, is the most general category for use in content analysis studies and was used in the present study (see chapter 4 for details of the process of finding a framework of analysis for the categories.)

Berelson defined content analysis and said this should be:

- *applied only to the syntatic and semantic dimensions of language.* The analysis then, is limited, to the 'manifest content' of the communication, rather than in terms of intentions or responses;
- *objective.* The categories should be defined so precisely that different analysts can apply them to the same body of content and secure the same results;
- *systematic.* All the relevant information is to be included, to eliminate partial or biased analysis of data; where data does not fit the analysis this is excluded from analysis. Additionally, the analysis should have a measure of general application;
- *quantifiable.* This is the most distinctive feature of content analysis, which distinguishes the procedure from ordinary reading. Of primary importance is the extent to which the analytic categories appear in the content, that is, the relative emphases and omissions.

This definition of content analysis helped to guide the present analysis, the findings of which are presented in chapter 4. (A summary of the experience of complying with Berelson's requirements is also detailed, see p.171.)

The qualitative analysis
Use of laddering diagrams The constructs and data gained from the laddering procedure were presented in diagrammatic form (after Allsop, 1980 and Hazelden, 1981).

Qualitative data cards and the development of a theory The taped transcripts of the laddered interviews were also subjected to qualitative analysis. Glaser and Strauss (1967) discussed the value of identifying conceptual categories and properties (elements of a category) which 'help the reader to see and hear vividly the people in the area under study'. They advocated the use of this approach 'in non-traditional areas where there is little or no technical literature'. Community psychiatric nursing falls into this latter description and, as such, it was opportune to subject the accounts given by the community psychiatric nurses during laddering to this type of analysis.

A review of the early texts and papers on managing qualitative data (Becker and Geer, 1960; Barton and Lazersfeld, 1969; Sieber, 1976), shows that they devote little attention to the problems of data analysis; this situation has been rectified in more recent papers (see Norris, 1981; Turner, 1981; Field and Morse, 1985; Chenitz and Swanson, 1986) which have been especially helpful.

The strategy used to handle the qualitative data in this study followed that suggested by Turner (1981) who used qualitative data category cards to sort the data into categories (figure 5). Turner (1981)

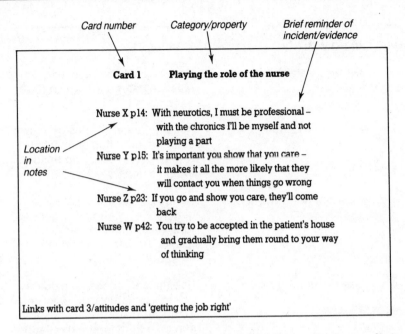

Figure 5 An example of a data category card for qualitative analysis

also elaborated a meticulous and systematic method of handling the practical elements of managing qualitative data, which consisted of a framework of nine stages (figure 6); it was formulated specifically for use in the development of grounded theory. The design of the present study was not faithful to a grounded approach, but using this framework, nevertheless, served the purpose of disciplining the researcher to examine the data closely in order to develop a theory which explained the 'process' of community psychiatric nursing. The method outlined by Turner was, therefore, followed in 'spirit' rather than to the letter. This first stage is elaborated at length, as it is the most 'opaque' step in the analysis. From transcription of taped material, Turner (1981) tentatively labelled the phenomena he was perceiving. He describes the process thus:

'I deal with the material paragraph by paragraph numbering the paragraphs for reference purposes. Starting with the first paragraph of the transcript I ask "What categories, concepts or labels do we need in order to describe or to account for the phenomenon discussed in this paragraph?" When I think of a label I note it down on a 5" x 8" file card, together with the number of the file and file the card. I then check whether further cards are needed to note significant phenomena referred to in this paragraph. I generate cards with titles of categories, until I am satisfied with my coverage of that paragraph, until I seem to have noted all of those features which are of significance to me, and then move on to the next paragraph. The labels used in this categorisation may be long

Stage	Main activity	Comment
1	Develop categories	Use the data available to develop labelled categories which fit the data closely
2	Saturate categories	Accumulate examples of a given category until it is clear what future instances would be located in this category
3	Abstract definitions	Abstract a definition of the category by stating in a general form the criteria for putting further instances into this category
4	Use the definitions	Use the definitions as a guide to emerging features of importance in further fieldwork, and as a stimulus to theoretical reflection
5	Exploit categories fully	Be aware of additional categories suggested by those you have produced, their inverse, their opposite, more specific and more general instances
6	Note, develop and follow-up links between categories	Begin to note relationships and develop hypotheses about the links between the categories
7	Consider the conditions under which the links hold	Examine any apparent or hypothesised relationships and try to specify the conditions
8	Make connections where relevant to existing theory	Build bridges to existing work at this state, rather than at the outset of the research
9	Use extreme comparisons to the maximum to test emerging relationships	Identify the key variables and dimensions and see whether the relationship holds at the extremes of these variables

(From Turner, 1981. Reproduced by kind permission of Elsevier Science Publishers)

Figure 6 Turner's nine-stage framework of qualitative analysis

winded, ungainly or fanciful at this stage and they may be formulated at any conceptual level which seems appropriate, but it is important that they should possess one essential property: as far as the researcher is concerned the label should fit the phenomena described in the data exactly. If the fit is not perfect, the words used should be changed and rechanged and adjusted until the fit is improved, for the value of the whole approach depends upon this goodness of fit as the basis of subsequent operations.'

Emphasising the use of techniques to handle the analysis of qualitative data tends to underplay the part of the researcher in the understanding of the data: the researcher brings her own theoretical and personal perspective to bear on the analytical process. As already mentioned, the community psychiatric background of the researcher will have influenced the study in different ways, and this comment is relevant to the interpretation of the interview data. The findings of this analysis are presented in chapter 4 and details of these have been published (Pollock, 1988).

The qualitative analysis was based on transcriptions from audio-tape recordings of the 'laddered interviews' and undertaken personally by the researcher. No resources were available to meet the heavy cost of professional help. Transcribing is considered a prerequisite to qualitative analysis (Field and Morse, 1985). Transcribing is a lengthy process and it took at least 10 to 12 hours to transcribe a 90-minute tape. This aspect of the analysis, then, involved a considerable investment of time.

The data from the first area was analysed before that of the second area, the reason being that data from the second site was used to confirm the findings of the first.

An innovative approach in the use of the method

The laddering procedure has been little used previously in research, but it provides a useful means of exploring the initial constructs. I had expected the nurses to give quite concise details about their work, but in fact they often gave lengthy details, volunteering plenty of information and examples to back up what they were saying. Often, the nurses would give two reasons together for being interested in particular information; these were both explored separately. Sometimes, the implications of the implicit pole came up spontaneously and it was unnecessary to repeat the question, 'Why?'. Often, the implications of the 'implicit pole' were not opposites of the other side of the ladder. Positive comments were made by the nurses about the procedure: 'It makes you think about things. You do this job and you do it normally without thinking what you are supposed to do. You've made me think why, and I've been surprised at some of the answers'. Continually asking why caused some nurses to wonder if they were unclear in their responses. Overall the nurses enjoyed talking about their work.

The laddering procedure took three to four hours, on average, to complete, although with some of the nurses it took longer. The laddering interviews were divided into two sessions depending on the demands of the nurses' work. I took notes, which were summaries of the content of the discussions; these did not distract the respondents, and helped me to clarify what I was interested in exploring. On occasions, my notes were my interpretations of what had been said rather than exact details; this inaccuracy of recording what was actually said was responsible at times for my asking for clarification of the wrong details. This shows how the demands of the interview situation affected the conversations and, at times, this meant that all constructs were not fully explored. Overall, the impression gained by the researcher was that the constructs were examined more fully than could have been achieved in normal conversation.

Taking a qualitative analysis to the data has shown that this method can be used more productively than it has been previously (Allsop, 1980; Hazelden, 1981); this approach to the analysis was more fruitful than using the more traditional quantitative analysis. Future research should exploit this method.

The personal questionnaire rapid scaling technique

The personal questionnaire rapid scaling technique (PQRST) was the method used for the 'outcome' part of the study. Personal question-naires were designed by Shapiro (1961) to measure patients' experiences, particularly symptoms and their improvement. The original method was revised by Mulhall (1971, 1976).

PQRST is capable of measuring beliefs, feelings and attitudes, and is specifically designed for evaluation of subjective experiences. PQRST is a type of questionnaire where, instead of questions being answered, a series of personalised statements are presented which the subject is asked to rate. The format differs from traditional questionnaires in that a booklet with answer sheets is used. The design of this booklet structures the answers and ensures that what is being measured is rated on an ordered metric scale (this is explained further below and illustrated in figures 7,8 and 10).

Advantages of the use of the PQRST
1.   The procedure has been validated in previous work (Ingham, 1965; Mulhall, 1976).
2.   The design is considered to be beneficial in reducing response bias.
3.   The logic of PQRST is that, in normal conversation, feelings are quantified by adjectival phrases and that these are closer to the normal process of describing quantity than is the necessary abstraction of using numbers or length of lines.

4. The descriptive terms used in the procedure have been extensively tested (Mulhall, 1978). These are: 'absolutely none', 'very little', 'little', 'moderate', 'considerable' and 'very considerable'.

5. All possible pairs of adjectives are employed, ensuring that the whole scale is used and that the central bias of traditional questionnaires is, hence, avoided.

6. The questionnaire is simple and rapid to use.

7. The scoring is similarly simple and expeditious, using a scoring key.

8. The adjectives are considered to be on an ordered metric scale; this is advantageous to the analysis and permits certain statistical manipulations to be undertaken on the data collected.

All of the above listed advantages positively influenced the choice of PQRST for use in the present study. Items 3 and 6 were particularly relevant to this study, which involved psychiatric patients and relatives, some of whom were also psychiatric patients.

Figures 7, 8 and 10 illustrate the PQRST procedure. Figure 7 shows the answer sheet; the concepts being assessed are listed on the right-hand side. These answer sheets are placed inside the PQRST booklet

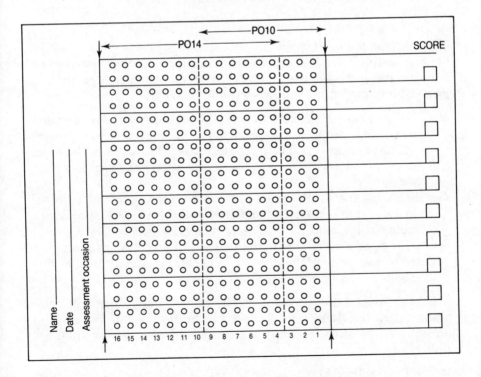

Figure 7   The answer sheet of the PQRST procedure

and respondents are presented with pairs of adjectives and asked which member of each pair comes closer to the concept being assessed. Figure 8 shows this stage of the procedure, using an example from Mulhall's work measuring symptom change.

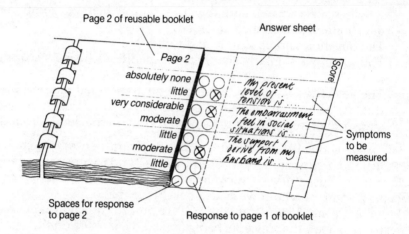

Figure 8   The PQRST booklet and answer sheet using Mulhall's (1968) format of symptoms

The construction of PQRST

Several methods are available for measuring psychological variables. For example, if the aim were to measure levels of anxiety experienced by a patient, any of the following might be used:

- a numerical scale from 1 to 7 in which 1 represents 'no anxiety' and 7 represents 'extreme anxiety'. In this case, the patient selects a number which characterises his present level of anxiety. The range of such a scale might be greater or less than seven;
- a straight line, with 'absence of anxiety' at one end and 'extreme anxiety' at the other. The patient marks the line at a point which indicates the amount of anxiety he experiences;
- a list of adjectives conveying degrees of anxiety, again ranging from absence to high intensity. The patient selects the adjective which seems appropriate.

These, and other related techniques, share the common assumption that there is an underlying continuum, in this case, of anxiety. While such methods are quick and easy to use they are unlikely to:

- reduce response bias, whether this is deliberate or inadvertant (see Cronbach, 1950);

- allow an assessment of reliability to be made;
- make allowances for the difficulty that some patients have in making abstractions which require an analogy to be made between the subjective intensity of the symptom and a numerical value or a length.

The PQRST is designed in such a way as to ensure that the whole of the scale is used; this is achieved by pairing each adjective with the adjacent one and to the one next to that (figure 9).

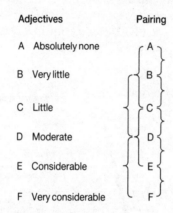

Figure 9　Adjective pairing in the PQRST

This arrangement of adjective pairs (nine in total) ensures that all possible discriminations are used, therefore eliminating bias. Each adjective location is ascribed a score:

```
   0   1   2   3   4   5   6   7   8   9
   A   |   B   |   C   |   D   |   E   |   F
```

Each set of adjectives used can be considered to form an ordinal scale. The interval between them is unknown and may, in fact, be different for different people. The scale cannot, therefore, be assumed to be an interval scale. The procedure assumes that the scale is ordered metrically. Within each pair of adjectives presented to the respondent, one implies greater magnitude than the other; an overall score is derived by counting the number of pairs in which the more intense adjective is chosen. If the lesser adjective is always chosen, the score is zero, if the greater is always chosen, the score is nine.

PQRST in the present study
The intention of the PQRST part of the present study was to examine the outcome of community psychiatric intervention. The main foci of

the study were, first, to find out how families of patients being visited by community psychiatric nurses perceived that community psychiatric nursing contact and, second, to see if, and to what extent, carers' problems and experiences of caring for a mentally-ill relative were helped by community psychiatric nursing intervention. Information about the patient's experience of the community psychiatric nursing contact was also collected.

Therefore, in the present study, instead of symptoms being listed (as referred to above), statements about the community psychiatric nurse, the service received or statements about patients' problems and the carers' experiences of caring were inserted (figure 10, and see tables 6, 7 and 8 in chapter 4). Details about how the statements were derived are detailed from p.107 onwards.

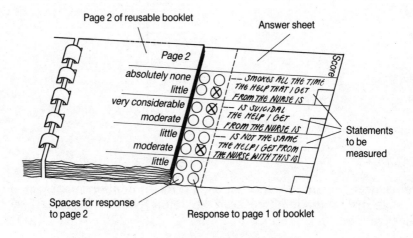

Figure 10   The PQRST booklet and answer sheet using
statements from the present study

Platt et al (1980) reviewed the research instruments which have been used in 'burden' research, and commented that the only single instrument which assessed the patient's disturbed behaviour and altered social performance, as well as assessing burden, was the 'family evaluation form' (FEF) developed by Spitzer et al (1971). Platt et al commented that this FEF was 'overly general and simplified'. Another researcher who used the FEF (see Kennedy and Hird, 1980) commented, in a personal communication to me, that this instrument was cumbersome to use. Platt et al (1980) proposed an alternative instrument be used to investigate 'burden' – the 'social behaviour assessment schedule' (SBAS) – the main advantage of this over previous techniques being that it allowed for clear separation and assessment, in one instrument, of patient disturbed behaviour and social performance and the adverse effect of this on the household. This tool, and those of other researchers investigating 'burden' (e.g. Grad and Sainsbury, 1968; Hoenig and Hamilton, 1969; Spitzer et al, 1971, Pai and Kapur, 1982; Platt et al, 1980; Mangen and Griffith, 1982b) took the form of semi-structured interviews which were often lengthy and which entailed ratings of carers' comments by the researcher/interviewer. These interviews were aimed at assessing the extent of burden experienced by carers.

The concern of this study was not to assess the extent of burden experienced by carers, but, rather, to focus on the relief given by the community psychiatric nurses for the different types of burden. Furthermore, this study wanted to look at the carers' view (not the researchers' interpretation of this), so previous tools used in burden research could not be directly applied. The PQRST seemed to be a method which could be used to achieve this aim. A further merit of PQRST as a method was that it could be easily used by carers.

Carers of patients being visited by community psychiatric nurses from both West and East Hospitals completed a 'family PQRST' (for a copy of these answer sheets, see appendix 6, Pollock, 1987). The 'family PQRST' comprised three sections (see figure 11). The first

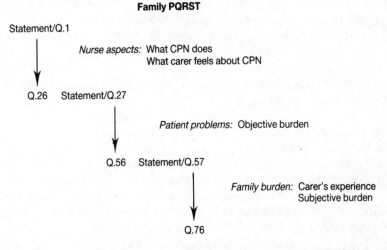

Family PQRST

Statement/Q.1

Nurse aspects: What CPN does
What carer feels about CPN

Q.26   Statement/Q.27

Patient problems: Objective burden

Q.56   Statement/Q.57

Family burden: Carer's experience
Subjective burden

Q.76

Figure 11 Diagram showing sections of the 'family PQRST'

section, questions 1–26, contained statements about what the community psychiatric nurse did and about the carers' perception of the community psychiatric nurse (this section was called 'nurse aspects'). The second section (called 'patient problems'), questions 27–56, contained statements about patient problems (described as 'objective burden' in the literature). Section three (called 'family burden'), questions 57–76, contained statements on carers' comments of their experience of caring (described in the literature as 'subjective burden'). The statements for section 1 were derived from the pilot study (see below). It proved difficult to gain statements about 'problems' from families in the pilot study; sections 2 and 3 of the PQRST, were, therefore, derived partly from relatives' comments during the pilot study and also from the past research on family burden (see p.107).

Two types of PQRST were used with patients. The 'home-visiting' PQRST was used with the patients of community psychiatric nurses of both East and West Hospitals. The 'day-care' PQRST was used only for the patients of East Hospital's nurses. The statements for the day-care and home-visiting questionnaires were all derived from the pilot study. Copies of the answer sheets can be found in appendixes 7 and 8, Pollock, 1987.

Respondents were asked to agree or disagree with the statements and then rate the community psychiatric nursing intervention on a scale of 'helpfulness'. In answer to each question, the respondents commented on how 'helpful' the nurses had been, choosing one of the range of descriptions: 'absolutely none', 'very little', 'little', 'moderate', 'considerable', and 'very considerable'. As explained above, for each question the respondent was forced to make a choice between two adjectives, and asked to tick the adjective that came nearest the 'true' rating (see figure 10 above).

Patients or families who were unable to complete the questionnaire on their own were asked the questions verbally. In these circumstances, the personal questionnaire, therefore, became a focused interview. As described by Denzin (1970), this is when 'certain types of information are desired from all respondents, but the particular phrasing of questions and their order are redefined to fit the characteristics of each respondent'. Lofland and Lofland (1984) call this focused interview a 'guided conversation'. The spontaneous comments about the community nursing service, voiced by patients and families during or after completion of the PQRST, were noted. As Blum (1970) has commented, conversation can be more relaxed and additional information can be gleaned after the more formal stage of interviewing and questionnaire-completion.

The information so collected contains both 'direct' and 'volunteered' statements. As elaborated by Becker and Geer (1960), the volunteered statements can be assumed to be representative of the patient's preoccupations and true feelings, whereas the directed statements have arisen as a result of the researcher's questions and biases. No attempt has been made to separate these comments, although, in retrospect, this would have been a valuable exercise.

Pilot study of the PQRST

The reasons for the pilot study
The PQRST is a research tool which has been previously used in research. The purpose of the pilot was not to refine the research tool itself but, rather, to test its use in the present study.

There were two main stages of this pilot study. The first was to acquire the list of statements to be used in the PQRST procedure. The second was to integrate these into the PQRST procedure and to pilot the method with community psychiatric nurses' patients and respective carers (see figure 2 above). Each of these stages is described below.

Statements to be included in the PQRST The aim of this stage was to gain statements which could be integrated into the PQRST format. In the first instance, members of self-help groups concerned with care of the mentally ill were approached to see if they were able to talk about their experiences and the difficulties of caring for a relative. The groups included were Scottish Association for Mental Health, Scottish Action on Dementia, the Alzheimer's Disease Society, the Schizophrenia Fellowship, and the Manic Depressives Association.

Members who were approached were organisers of these associations, all of whom were carers of mentally-ill people. They were informed that my research interest was the effect on relatives of caring for someone who is mentally ill, and that I would like to interview them about their experiences. In this way, it was hoped to acquire statements on objective and subjective burden. The respondents were able to talk about their difficulties, and especially focused on practical difficulties with which they were faced: the patient's wandering or keeping himself to himself, not coping with the DHSS/money, or smoking too much, were commonly mentioned.

Secondly, 24 patients and their respective carers, clients of East Hospital's community psychiatric nurses, were interviewed in their own homes. These patients/carers – three from each community psychiatric nurse – were not included in the main study; they were chosen after the subjects in the main study had been selected (see pp.77 and 80) and on the basis that they reflected a variety of frequency of contacts. The aim of these interviews was to gain information about the 'process' of community psychiatric nursing from patients and families. Patients and carers were asked to tell me about their contact with the community psychiatric nurse; the carers were asked to describe how the nurses helped with particular problems. In this way, it was hoped to generate statements which could be included in the PQRST answer sheets for use in the main study.

Only four patients in the pilot study refused to be interviewed. Of the remainder, patients were seen by the community psychiatric nurse either at a day centre (eight), or at home (12); eight had had contact at the day centre but were presently seen at home. Comments about the community psychiatric nursing contact varied depending on the setting in which this took place. On this basis, two different types of PQRST were devised: one for patients who attended the day centre and one for patients visited at home. Patients in the main study would fill in the PQRST which described the present contact with the community psychiatric nurse; if patients were receiving both home and day care the 'home-visiting' PQRST was completed.

Interviews took place with 14 carers, and three others refused to make comment. Seven patients refused me permission to contact their relatives. Information about the carers' view of 'process' was obtained, but it was difficult to gain information from the relatives about problems or about how the community psychiatric nurses helped them with their experiences. The carers who did provide descriptions of the reality of caring did so in the terms most meaningful to them (for example, 'I can never tell what so-and-so will do next'). These descriptions used less jargon than those found in the literature (using the previous example, the literature would have said the patient was 'unpredictable'). As far as was possible, statements in the PQRST used a minimum of jargon in an attempt to make the exercise as meaningful as possible to the carers.

Having failed to elicit an extensive list of 'problems' from the carers, the literature on burden was consulted again in order to gain a comprehensive list of 'burdensome' factors which could be used in the PQRST (see references above). The resulting 'family PQRST', therefore, included comments from the carers in the pilot interviews, plus items from literature sources. The final list of statements was endorsed by the members of the voluntary organisations mentioned above to check that no major 'problem' had been missed out.

Use of the PQRST procedure The second stage of the pilot study consisted of using the proposed PQRST and answer sheets with patients and carers. Included in this stage of the pilot study were 10 of the patient/carer pairs who had been previously interviewed. The procedure was successfully completed by patients and carers; it took longer than expected and the repetitious nature of the procedure was commented on by some. On the answer sheets, beside the statements, there was a square for the score (see figure 7): this was distracting to respondents, as was the fact that previous responses became visible as progress was made through the booklet (see figure 8). Feedback from this stage of the pilot about the specific statements resulted in some of these being omitted from the main study. A major modification was a clearer separation of the activity of the nurse, or problem experienced by the carer (the statement), and the question to be answered ('the help that the visiting nurse gave me was . . .').

Although the purpose of the pilot run was to gain information for use in the PQRST, it highlighted other issues surrounding 'doing research'. In particular it made me focus on aspects of the process of interviewing patients/carers in their own homes and on my role as a researcher. These interpersonal factors are mentioned here because it is acknowledged that they may have had a biasing effect on the study.

The process of interviewing I introduced myself, in the pilot, as a university student, learning about research by doing a study on community psychiatric nursing; I said that I had got the patient's name from the community psychiatric nurses in East Hospital. I deliberately intended to be seen as separated from the parent hospital service. This seemed to cause two problems.

First, the effect of my introduction was that respondents asked me various questions: some respondents asked about my employer, why I was doing the study and what was I going to do with the resulting information. I said that I would be writing the project up as part of my degree. Other respondents were explicitly worried about whether or not the community psychiatric nursing service would be adversely affected as a result of the study. This, of course, was an extremely difficult question to answer as no researcher can predict the effects of the research. All that I could reply was that my intention was to examine community psychiatric nursing because this was a developing speciality.

Second, my introduction seemed to cause respondents to reply to my questions in vague terms, e.g. 'her type of problem' or 'nerve troubles', and there was a general reluctance on the part of respondents to discuss details of difficulties or of community psychiatric nursing contact. Because of this, I decided to tell respondents (after the fifth interview) that I had a community psychiatric nursing background. This seemed to help patients and relatives to verbalise their problems; maybe they made (positive) assumptions about my reactions and professional understandings. This may also, however, have had the (negative) effect of making some patients/carers less critical of a service with which (they assumed) I had sympathies. I also did this in the main study.

The lack of flow of discussion may have been compounded by two other factors. First and foremost, I arrived with the patients/carers unannounced and without any warning. This may have resulted in a general suspicion about my credentials and motives which may have been reflected in a reluctance to talk to me. This could have been remedied by my explaining the study and returning when respondents had time to think; lack of time on my part prevented this (see also p.111). I wrote to two people in the pilot study giving warning that I was going to visit on a certain date and time, and giving a phone number to contact me on if this was inconvenient. These two respondents were extremely anxious about my mode of contact and I, therefore, decided that it was better to deal with these anxieties at the time rather than to let people worry.

The second factor which may have discouraged communication (particularly that of a sensitive nature) was that, on arrival at houses, I immediately started questioning and note-taking. This, of course, reduced eye contact and did little to encourage communication and rapport.

Some respondents specifically said that they did not want their names mentioned anywhere in the study and stated that they did not want their case histories identified.

Others were concerned about how I had gained access to their names and addresses; they were alarmed that I had also gained information about their illness or personal details. I, in fact, only needed and used details of names and addresses for this part of the study, and I informed the respondents of this. (I did, actually, have access to case-notes and Kardexes which contained personal information which I did not access, but I did not share this with the respondents.) I told these respondents that the names and addresses had not been given readily, and that permission to do the research had been given by the Hospital Management Committee, the Area Ethics Committee and the parent hospital's consultants and community psychiatric nurses. I decided to inform all participants in the main study about these details, and to stress that all questionnaire answers would be anonymous.

In the pilot study, there were three occasions when both carer and family were in the house together. I had intended to interview patients first and then ask if I could approach the relatives as well, but, in reality, to do this would have imposed an artificial separation on the situation. There were also practical difficulties when the carer was the more vocal and outspoken member of a couple. I decided, therefore, to 'play it by ear' and answer whichever questions came up, and set out to cover the specific research questions to each as intended. I acknowledge that the presence of the other person may have inhibited the respondent's replies.

This experience did, however, raise the question of whether or not I would give the PQRST questionnaires to both together if this situation arose in the main study. I decided to do so, especially as the written format of the PQRST made it less inhibiting to the carer or patient.

Visiting patients and families at home was extremely time-consuming; often I had to make return visits, either because no-one was in or in order to see the relative. Commonly, addresses were difficult to find and, in some cases, the addresses were out of date.

The pilot study made me aware of all these difficulties, many of which could not be resolved. For reasons of economy in relation to money and time, patients and carers in the same areas were visited on planned days.

As mentioned above, I told respondents of my community psychiatric nursing background. Whether or not as a result of this, some patients and relatives mentioned their mental health or situation to me and asked for advice; for example, one lady said she felt shaky and was it her drugs? Another said that the community psychiatric nurse was trying to get her to go to the day centre and did I agree? A relative asked if 'the patient' would get better.

This is a situation similar to that described by other nurse researchers using the method of 'observation' (Pearsall, 1965). Pearsall talks of interviewing as a major ingredient of participant observation and commented, 'Tensions may be expected between some of the norms associated with research and their almost opposite counterparts in nursing practice – between disinterested observation and interested action . . .'. I was faced with this dilemma – should I respond to the interviewees and PQRST respondents in my 'nursing' role or in that of 'researcher?' I decided to avoid slipping into the 'interested action' role of the nurse; if, wearing my 'nursing hat', I was worried about a patient or relative, I would contact the parent hospital.

Also, in an attempt to maintain the role of researcher, that described by Blenkner (1950) as the 'investigative role' rather than that of 'primarily helping', I tried to make the interviews formal. I refused to have coffee, for instance – I found that 'having coffee' made the situation less formal and that respondents asked more questions, not only about me personally and professionally, but also about what I thought of East Hospital, the treatment and the community psychiatric nurses there. This is a small point, but one which I considered: I tried to be as consistent as possible in my approach to all patients and carers in an attempt to reduce any bias into the interviews, and this stance was taken throughout the main study.

Analysis of the data from the PQRST method

Using a scoring template, the method of PQRST enabled conversion of the adjectives used by respondents into a score of 0 ('absolutely no help') to 9 ('a very considerable help'), as discussed above. The number of responses in each horizontal row of the answer sheet were counted and checked to see if they were consecutively numbered; if so, the score was written in the box of the answer sheet. This method was fast and was facilitated by the format of the answer sheet. Scores were then inserted into a data file (see appendix 9, Pollock, 1987).

The numerical information obtained from the PQRST was

subjected to statistical manipulation using the non-parametric statistical packages available on the university mainframe computer (Siegel, 1956). The Statistical Package for the Social Sciences mentioned above had been updated by the time of analysis of the PQRST data, and the updated version, called SPSSx (Nie, 1983) was used for this part of the study.

The responses to each statement on the PQRST were examined using descriptive statistics. This gave an indication of the types of problem with which the families had to cope, gave an indication of the families' experience of the community psychiatric nursing service and provided a measure of how helpful the nurses actually were. Standard chi-square tests of association were also used, to see if there were specific aspects of the nurse or carer that affected helpfulness. Variables examined included the sex and age of the carer and the case-loads and visiting frequency patterns of the nurses. Scattergrams were compiled and multiple regression analysis was attempted.

The PQRST proved to be a useful means of exploring nurse helpfulness. There were difficulties ultimately in interpreting the scores (see chapter 4): if a nurse was rated as 'helpful' it was unclear why this was the case (and vice versa). The scores would have been more meaningful had they been linked with other data, patient history or illness, or age of carer, for example.

4 | The results

In this chapter, the results of the study are presented. There are four sections: the nurses', patients' and carers' views of community pyschiatric nursing and details of the goals of the service. The chapter ends with a summary of the study, with a review of the findings and limitations of the work.

THE NURSES' VIEW OF THE SERVICE

The repertory grid technique and laddering procedure provided the opportunity to explore the work of the community psychiatric nurses. In this section, the findings of this part of the study are presented. First, the 'elements' used by the nurses are detailed and discussed. Most of this section is devoted to presentation of the results of the qualitative analysis of the laddered interviews. It was hoped that this would provide qualitative data on the way in which a small number of CPNs work and, in particular, focus on the nurses' work with carers.

The element lists produced by the nurses

During the preliminary periods of observation, the community psychiatric nurses in each study area were interviewed and asked to describe their work. Each community psychiatric nurse produced a list of patient types with whom they were in contact and activities which they specifically did, e.g. 'I run a self-help group for depressed women'; 'I organise an injection clinic for schizophrenic patients'; 'I liaise with other professionals and attend hospital Kardex discussions'. These descriptions could be summarised as 'task-centred' definitions of community psychiatric nursing. Carr et al (1980), for instance, defined six aspects of the role of the community psychiatric nurse, and Butterworth and Skidmore (1981) proposed various 'treatment approaches' available to psychiatric nurses dealing with the mentally ill in the community. None of these frameworks was described by the nurses when initially asked to describe their work.

113

Before detailing the results of the qualitative analysis, the differences in the 'element list' (see appendix V) used for the two study areas will be examined and commented on. Although the work patterns of the community psychiatric nurses were not systematically studied, differences in the work patterns of the nurses can be deduced from the varied descriptions given in the 'element list'.

Nine out of the 15 patient descriptions were similar: 'depot patient', 'consultant referral', 'at-risk patient', 'depressive patient', 'demented patient', 'new referral', 'GP referral' and 'chronic patient'. 'Home assessment' visits described by the nurses attached to West Hospital coincided with the East Hospital nurses' description of 'requested visits', although the nurses attached to West Hospital would do a home assessment at the request of professionals other than hospital staff. There were, therefore, in total, 10 elements produced that were similar in the two community psychiatric nursing services.

The other elements described by the community psychiatric nurses differed. The East Hospital nurses had two labels describing patients in terms of medication given; this reflected an emphasis, evident in East Hospital nurses' work, on administering and delivering medication. East Hospital nurses also took blood samples to measure 'lithium' levels, an activity not undertaken by the nurses attached to West Hospital. This preoccupation with provision of medication was less evident in the West Hospital nurses' work.

Both areas saw patients in terms of GP referrals, but West Hospital nurses also described patients in terms of 'which agency' referred, e.g. health visitor or social work referral; this reflected the open referral system operated by the West Hospital nurses. The East Hospital nurses only accepted consultant referrals. This, combined with the descriptions of 'outpatient', 'requested visit' (request from wards or day centre staff to visit at weekends), 'physically ill' and 'inpatient' could suggest that this reflected a hospital and medical orientation in the practice of the East Hospital nurses. The West Hospital nurses were GP-attached and were less involved with the parent hospital (see chapter 3). Examination of the constructs produced by each community psychiatric nurse (the findings of which are summarised below) suggested that the West Hospital nurses also had a more 'problem orientated' view of their patients.

The West Hospital nurses described 'anxiety-management patients', 'crisis calls' and 'social visits'; these were not as relevant for the East Hospital nurses' work. It could be deduced that West Hospital nurses saw themselves more as a crisis- and anxiety-management service than did the East Hospital nurses. Figure 12 shows that West Hospital nurses produced more 'description of treatment' constructs than did those from East Hospital. The element list also mirrors this difference, and the West Hospital nurses described patients in terms of treatment offered, e.g. 'home assessment', 'crisis call' and 'social visits'.

The element lists resulted from discussions with the nurses, and the final list is representative of agreed descriptions of the community psychiatric nurses as a group. This does not reflect the range of descriptions used by the nurses in practice (see p.137). Each element list gives descriptions used by all the community psychiatric nurses. Some of the East Hospital nurses described 'emergency call-outs' and 'patients on support and maintenance only' which appear comparable to the elements 'crisis calls' and 'social visits' respectively described by the West Hospital nurses. There was almost total agreement by the West Hospital nurses of the element list; this could suggest that they carried out similar types of work. The different grades and work settings of the East Hospital nurses may have produced the variety there.

Although beyond the scope of the present study, it would be fascinating to find out what was responsible for the differences in the emphasis of the community psychiatric nursing services. Why were the nurses attached to the West Hospital more problem orientated and those in the East Hospital more medication orientated? Why did West Hospital accept referrals from a wide range of agencies and East Hospital only from doctors? These questions arose out of the present study and were not explored further.

The work of the community psychiatric nurses

Summary of the qualitative analysis
These data explain how community psychiatric nurses make community psychiatric nursing work. The work of community psychiatric nursing can be usefully compared to that involved in a theatre production. In the theatre, there is a play with a plot which is conveyed through the parts played by the characters. In the face of production limitations (size of theatre, costs and time constraints, for example), and the demands of sponsors, audience, theatre critics and others in the company, the characters make use of the stage props and 'get the show on the road'.

The community psychiatric nurses can be likened to the characters in a play whose title is 'The provision of a community psychiatric nursing service', the plot being the provision of individualised care. Similar to the production limitations in the theatre, the community psychiatric nurses have limited care options and resources, and are faced with the varied demands of patients, carers and situations, other specialists and the bureaucracy. Yet, the nurses have to produce the best match of needs to resources. Maintaining the theatrical analogy, the nurses have to use what props they have on the stage, not to 'get the show on the road', but to make the community pyschiatric nursing service work.

Unlike a theatrical production, however, community psychiatric nurses do not appear to have an overall director controlling the work; neither are there guidelines which limit or define practice. This results in individual community psychiatric nurses establishing their own *modus operandi* and defining their own work practices.

Two major themes pervade this account of the work of the community psychiatric nurses. Firstly, the nurses 'juggle resources'. Secondly, they continually seek to legitimise their work and justify the care given. Both of these aspects of the work have emerged because the nurses' expressed ideology of providing 'individualised' care (care tailored to the needs of individual patients and their carers) has been impossible to sustain in the face of finite resources.

The ideology of individualised care

Traditional psychiatry and psychiatric theories and models (see chapter 2) have been criticised because they focus on the 'individual'; this approach renders individually-experienced difficulties as individual problems, regardless of their cause (Penfold and Walker, 1983; Banton et al, 1985). Penfold and Walker, for instance, have stated that psychiatry takes:

> 'the "individual" as both the *unit of study* and as the *unit of meaning*. This can be characterised as merely an extension of the Western ideology of "individualism". It is more accurately understood as a function of the way that "the social and economic organization of society generates typical situations for people to endure as *individuals* because they have no power to change them and do not see them as matters which can be changed." It is this assumption that results in the further assumption that individually experienced difficulties are indeed individual problems, regardless of cause.'

Despite this criticism, the principle of respect for the 'individual' is widely described as being the central principle of the caring professions (see Downie and Telfer, 1980). Furthermore, in recent years, the trend in nursing has been away from telling the patient what is best for him and what he should do, and towards involving him in the decision-making process. The 'nursing process', an approach to care which emphasises that each person is an individual who has needs and problems peculiar to him, and that the patient has a right to have a say in what is done for him, is testimony to the importance placed on care of the 'individual' in contemporary nursing (Aggleton and Chalmers, 1986). Community psychiatric nursing is no different in this respect, and one of the notable aspects of the data collected in this study was the expression of an ideology of 'individualised' care by the community psychiatric nurses.

The work, as described by the community psychiatric nurses, and the resources used (and often created by) the community psychiatric nurses, were 'patient-focused'. The nurses claimed to plan care on an 'individual' basis and talked about getting to know the patients as 'individuals'. They emphasised that this was intrinsic to the implementation of therapy and a prerequisite to any activities of the community psychiatric nurses. The importance of this became apparent because, before they committed themselves verbally to the researcher about what they would do in relation to specific situations or patients, the nurses stressed the need to 'get to know the patients'.

Psychiatric nurses obviously have 'to get to know the patients'; they have to talk to patients and gather information in order to do their jobs adequately. This is the initial data gathering or 'assessment' stage of the 'nursing process', the prevalent prescriptive model used by many nurses. In addition to this, the community psychiatric nurses have to 'get to know the carers'. This is particularly important in the community setting as the nurses have less control of the situation than they do when caring for patients in hospitals. All the community psychiatric nurses constantly referred to 'getting to know the patients' and 'getting to know the relatives'.

Developing and building relationships Three other references in the data lent support to the notion of the nurses providing 'individualised' care. Firstly, the nurses spoke at length of 'building and developing relationships' with 'individual' patients, and referred to this as part of the process of 'getting to know individuals'. 'Building relationships' is a generally accepted premise on which psychiatric nursing is based (see chapter 2), as Burgess and other authors have commented. Burgess (1981), for instance, has stated:

'Feeling responsible for a person in terms of being involved with his well-being and by helping him to reach for mutually agreed upon goals is in reality caring for the patient. As the patient works with the nurse on goals for recovery, he will use the nurse's humanness and strength to build back his own resources. In giving of oneself, through one's own uniqueness, coupled with an attitude of being genuinely interested in the patient and trying to understand and help him, the nurse will find developing the fundamentals of relating with the patient.'

The comments of one community psychiatric nurse in this study (Hamish) summarised that of many others:

'We can't really help unless we know what is going on. We build a relationship with them and get to know them. They get to know us and trust us.'

The 'getting to know' behaviours of the individual nurses varied from having cups of tea, 'to break down barriers', to talking to patients, giving medication and collecting specimens of urine or blood (East Hospital nurses only). As nurse Adam explained:

'If we have taken someone on in the community, we have a fair bit of work initially, just the main investigations for one thing – going in and out the house, you find out who is who, just because you are doing the creatinine clearance, lithium levels or different things; you are still getting to know them, no matter which way it goes.'

Schwartz and Shockley (1956) also found that the nurses undertook activities along with the development of interpersonal relations between patients and nurses. They said:

'We believe this aspect [interpersonal relations] to be crucial in bringing about patient improvement. Whatever a nurse is doing with the patient – bathing him, feeding him, giving him medication, playing games with him or sitting talking with him – she is maintaining a relationship with him. We need to know more about these nurse/patient interactions and their effects on patients.'

Some information has been provided (see below) on the patient's perception of the community psychiatric nurse interaction, and it suggests that different patients found different activities helpful.

'Getting to know the relatives' was also acknowledged by the community psychiatric nurses as an important part of their work. As one nurse (Jock) said:

'You've got to get on good terms with the relatives. If they don't like you, you won't even get into the house. That will be it. I wouldn't want that. After all, I am the visitor going into the home.'

The strategy of 'showing care'   This brings us to the second reference in the data which supports the notion of the community nurses holding an ideology of individualised care, that is, the nurses spoke of 'showing that they cared'. This was a specific strategy used by the community psychiatric nurses which enabled them, as shown in the above quotation, to gain access to patients' homes.

Unlike the hospital situation, provision of care in the home environment allows patients to maintain social roles (see chapter 2). In the community situation, patients are not the passive recipients of care (as has been described in the hospital situation by Freidson, 1970; Penfold and Walker, 1983; Banton et al, 1985), and nurses are the guests of patients. The roles of the patient and the nurse are much more equal than when care is provided in the institutional setting. This affects the work of community psychiatric nurses in that they have to work at 'getting accepted' in the patient's home. The nurses referred to the work of gaining access at different levels, to gain acceptance in the home in the first place, secondly, to make it clear why they are there and what they can offer, and finally, to maintain that acceptance in order to be allowed to continue gaining entry to the patient's house. Examples showing each of these levels are listed below:

'With recent contacts you are trying to be accepted and you have to establish rapport.' (Adam)

'It's important to ask patients about aspects of their daily life; that makes sure they know you are trying to help and are sympathetic to their problems.' (Colin)

'You want to bring people round to your way of thinking but you've got to play it carefully and not tread on anyone's toes; they'll just not have you back.' (Bert)

'Showing that you care', then, was a strategy used by the nurses to 'gain access'. The nurses talked about the importance of 'showing you care' by 'playing the role of the nurse'. Both of these notions were inextricably linked, and repeated mention was made by the nurses about expectations, held by both patients and carers, of their behaviour as nurses and professionals. This is illustrated in the following extract:

'I have to be on guard to remain constructive, keep my feelings to myself. I get superconfrontive and very irritated and that is no way to be – I've got to play the caring role.' (Frank)

The idea of playing the role of the nurse may suggest that the nurses are in some way putting on an 'act'. This behaviour could, alternatively, be interpreted as a crucial part of the work of the psychiatric nurse. Nurses are taught about the importance of using empathy, warmth and a non-judgmental approach in order to develop relationships and facilitate communications (Rogers, 1957). 'Showing you care' and 'playing the role of the nurse' may be the nurses' umbrella terms for the activities which are evidence of the theory proposed by Rogers being put into practice.

The nurses had to demonstrate that they cared; this was despite being able to offer little help in some cases. They seemed to be successful in achieving this by asking questions, listening, showing interest and simply by 'being available'. The nurses considered these behaviours, at times combined with the provision of what could be described as 'gestures of concern', as sufficient action to 'show they cared':

'I'll always say, "I am a phone-call away, get in touch". We have a card saying "Community nursing services"; I'll leave that on my first visit – it's fairly standard practice.' (Kevin)

'Caring is not necessarily regular visits, it's being available, isn't it? It can take the form of a phone-call or having someone call and ask for a visit every three or four months. Time and time again, you find the relatives have not been dealt with or told things. What we are really into now is not following up but going along and introducing ourselves, leaving a phone number, being a known face.' (Lester)

By using the strategy of 'showing that they cared', the nurses were able to manage crises, provide early treatment and prevent hospitalisation. This strategy was used by the nurses to achieve desirable outcomes and was advantageous to the nurses at a practical level. Preventing hospitalisation was a frequently-cited goal of the work of the nurses, and one way of achieving this was to 'manage crisis' and 'implement early treatment'.

By 'showing that they cared', the nurses were able to keep the channels of communication open to ensure that they could be contacted in the event of crisis:

> 'You want to turn up if you know something is going on (an illness or bereavement) to show you care. That makes it all the more likely that they will come to you when things go wrong.' (Adam)

Crisis management is considered to be an ideal type of treatment for psychiatric patients (Caplan, 1964) and 'crisis intervention' (see chapter 2) has been described as an approach to care which is especially useful for community psychiatric nurses (Pullen and Gilbert, 1979a,b; Simmons and Brooker, 1986; Ratna, undated). This approach is clearly discernible from the data, as evidenced by the following excerpt:

> 'The sooner we get there, the sooner we see the patient in crisis, and they are more likely to tell us what happened to them, and be more aware of their own feelings and how they cannot cope. It is important for us to see them like that . . . we want to keep people at home. Home is best. They'll have a crisis at home, and, hopefully, they can get over the crisis and stay at home; that is part of our job.' (Graham)

By 'showing they cared', the nurses ensured that they would be called to patients should there be a crisis of any kind; this, in turn, was preferred by the nurses because they considered this time to be vital as regards patient change and improvement. This approach also enabled the nurses to provide early treatment.

The community psychiatric nursing literature underlines the importance of 'implementing early and quick treatment' where the term 'early treatment' refers to treatment of mental illness at an early stage before admission to hospital is indicated (MacDonald, 1972; Leopoldt, 1979a,b). This was relevant to the nurses in the present study. Kevin, for example, stated, 'If someone is "going off" or "going down", we want to know about it. If we can stop them, it will avoid re-admission and starting all over again. I would prefer to be contacted'. The community psychiatric nurses also talked of 'situational crises' as incidents which were handled in a particular way which focused on stress management and aimed at avoidance of hospital admission.

Reduction in hospital admission rates has been accredited to the work of community psychiatric nurses (Warren, 1971; Corrigan and Soni, 1977; Pullen, 1980), and the community psychiatric literature suggests that preventing admission to hospital is considered desirable (Stobie and Hopkins, 1972a, b; Harker et al, 1976). There was some suggestion from the data that the nurses were judged by their ability to prevent readmission, and this, in itself, was evidence which proved that the nurse 'cared', as the following extract shows:

> 'From the patient's point of view it [hospitalisation] sets them back . . . for my own credibility if they [the patient and carer] are going to have faith in you, you have to show some results. If you can, avoid anything like that [hospitalisation]. You have got to rely on the patient having confidence in you; if you establish that sort of rapport, they will get in touch as they trust you, and I work to prevent readmission – I show I care.' (Kevin)

Keeping patients out of hospital, however, depends on many factors, and not just on community psychiatric nursing contact. Goldberg and Huxley (1980) have shown that GPs play a vital role in the identification of mental illness and referral to the psychiatric services. West Hospital nurses' close links with GPs and acceptance of direct GP referrals suggest that this factor is acknowledged by that service.

Society's ability to tolerate non-productive people visible in the community has an important bearing on whether admission is considered (Hawks, 1975). The nurses referred to this as influencing their work:

> 'I want to prevent readmission especially if there is a "neighbour problem" – they may be a bit wary of the chap next door. The more admissions the patient has, the more social pressure there is to result in long-term care.' (Jock)

The family's ability and capacity to continue caring for a mentally-ill relative also influences the decision to admit to hospital. The nurses of both services referred to the latter two factors as having a bearing on the decision of whether to admit or not, and stated that they would not 'prevent admission to hospital *at all costs*'.

Psychiatric hospitals have, of course, in the past, been called 'asylums' (meaning 'sanctuary' or 'place of safety'), reminding us that the institution has qualities that recommend its use. A benefit of hospital admission has been pointed out by Cumming and Cumming (1957): they found that admission serves the purpose of 'preservation of the sane'. This was also the finding of Tizard and Grad (1961) who found that the domestic life of families was improved as a result of admission of a mentally-ill relative to hospital.

Both East and West Hospital community psychiatric nurses used hospital admission in this way; demented patients, in particular, regularly came into hospital for 'holiday admissions' to give their carers relief. Another reason given by the nurses for admitting patients was to allow 24-hour assessment, which would enable more information to be gained about patient behaviour (and, hence, more appropriate care to be given). Day and night care was considered desirable by the nurses for some patients who were considered 'at risk'. These were usually patients who lived on their own and were 'at risk of neglecting themselves', or patients described as 'impulsive, who may do something silly, like taking tablets ... they create anxiety in us; we look at how they have coped with crisis in the past; if they have taken an overdose we would be extremely anxious.'

Most of the work of the nurses, however, was to do with preventing hospitalisation. The avoidance of producing 'institutionalised' patients was the most common reason given by the nurses for preventing hospitalisation. Other reasons given by the nurses in the study included avoiding disruption of family life (see above), and avoiding labelling and stigma (see p.137). 'Caring' reasons, then, were given by the nurses to account for the emphasis of the work being done on prevention of hospitalisation. These reasons supported the notion of the work being focused on individuals and reinforced the nurses' approach of 'showing that they cared'.

The strategy of promoting patient independence   A third theme in the data lent support to the nurses carrying out 'individualised' care. This was the emphasis in the nurses' comments on helping individuals to be autonomous and capable of planning their own lives without professional help. The nurses talked about 'getting the patient independent'. The adoption of this rationale was central to the work of the community psychiatric nurses and emerged as a major reason for community psychiatric nursing intervention. The nurses referred to this by using different phrases: patients must 'stand on their own two feet'; 'run their lives for themselves'; 'act like adults'; 'make their own decisions'; 'have a realistic sense of responsibility'; 'be helped to cope with everyday aspects of living'; 'learn to adapt to change'. These phrases appear similar to lay attitudes to mental illness, where sufferers are told 'to pull themselves together'. One could conclude, therefore, that nurses used a 'lay' or common-sense approach to patients (as also found by Altschul, 1972a). An alternative interpretation of the nurses' rationale is that 'getting the patients independent' is seen as a crucial aspect of their 'caring' function and as intrinsic to their professional ideology of 'individualised' care.

It is perhaps at one remove from analysis of the data, but it is worth commenting in passing that this sentiment of 'maintaining independence' closely mirrors one strand of contemporary political philosophy; see chapter 2 for a discussion of how this is influencing the development of 'community care'. The data do not suggest that the nurses were taking this specific approach out of any particular political allegiance, but, rather, because of their concern for the welfare of the patient. However, the ambiguous nature of the approach is noteworthy.

The varied vocabularies used by the community psychiatric nurses suggest that different stances were taken with different patients; these ranged from a dictatorial, prescriptive role to a facilitative, supportive one. 'Getting patients independent' was a 'caring' way of describing work that was aimed at getting patients' deviant behaviour to conform to that sanctioned by society.

Individual nurses' modi operandi The notion of providing 'individual care' was confirmed by the finding that similar situations appeared to be treated differently by individual community psychiatric nurses within the same community psychiatric nursing services studied. The following excerpts show the differing interpretations:

> 'Isolation − I feel this is really a curse of this age; there are too many people without good neighbours. I feel that, with all the people out working, there is not as much caring; many people are totally isolated and I am the only person who looks in. I can be the only person that these people see. My job is to try and rectify that if I can, try to encourage them to get out or at least offer some social stimulation and company . . .' (Ivan)

> 'Those that are lonely and isolated, for instance − I know [a colleague] visits them. She has some she has seen for ages and she has some she has cut down on; but it's the weekly cups of tea that make me feel bad and angry. I don't think that is what you are paid for. And it is not an ideal world − there are a lot of people that you could be visiting occasionally, but the reality of it is that there are an awful lot more acute and distressed people around . . .' (Jock)

The examples chosen deliberately cover the same topic in order to facilitate discussion of the relevant issues. Other topics could have been used, for example, bathing patients, giving depot injections or transporting patients, to name but a few. These demonstrate the conflicting views, even within the same services, about the specific work of community psychiatric nursing.

It was apparent from the data that each community psychiatric nurse developed his own *modus operandi*. The nurses emphasised that each patient's and family's needs were different, that each, therefore, had to be assessed and that programmes had to be developed to cater for specific needs. Many descriptions of care demonstrated that the nurses considered 'assessment' to be a prerequisite to care provision, yet no formal assessment tools were used (e.g. Barker, 1986). One of the nurses in the study stated:

> 'If they were asking for an assessment, I'd do it on a "one-off' basis, but I would not get involved unless I had the GP's OK. It may be just a discussion and I'd say the approach that I would take.' (Kevin)

Some of the nurses talked of 'goal-setting', 'target-setting' and providing 'time-limited' packages of care. These strategies helped the nurses to structure the work, as demonstrated in the following excerpt:

'I'd set limited goals about keeping his health, making sure that physically and mentally he was as well as he could be, not at risk in his environment. I would not aim for employment for psychotics. I don't like setting too high a goal because, if I don't reach it, I feel bad within myself.' (Kevin)

Each nurse developed his own strategies and set of guidelines; there was considerable variation in the treatments which the nurses offered, and each nurse had particular preferences for certain tactics. Comparison of the following comments make this point:

'I'm not for tapes. Most of my colleagues use the relaxation tapes. I'm not for them – a busy mum with kids has not got time to set aside to relax. I'd just talk. I'd maybe set small targets, going to the shops, say. I would not give tapes. The information sheet is OK. I'll give it to them to read; if they do, I may give them a tape. It often makes the nurses feel better giving tapes over – it is an instant cure.' (Kevin)

'I have guidelines for people with panic attacks. I do four visits for assessment and background, that sort of thing, then we both (patient and nurse) decide if it is worthwhile. That is my way of trying to avoid the long-term dependency thing and also my feeling that I have to cure everyone. I think everyone should have that sort of "whatever" – when they look back and say where are we going? – otherwise it is a waste of time.' (Lester)

Although the nurses talked about working out care on an individual basis, and gave the impression of carrying out individually-tailored programmes, it might also be argued from the data that lack of resources was an important factor in care provision. The data showed that concern for the individual (patient and/or carer) was not necessarily the guiding premise, and much of the way in which community psychiatric nurses went about their work was to do with using and stretching the available resources to the limit.

Juggling resources
The nurses saw themselves as specialists and as a scarce resource. At times, the nurses felt 'pressured' to take action, as evidenced by the following comments: 'We are supposed to be a specialist type of nursing and able to give a diagnosis back to the GP of whether the person is psychiatrically ill or not' (Bert). Sometimes they felt they had no choice but to respond to the demands made of them, as shown in the next comment:

'The non-psychotics are easier to work with because the work is time limited. Because there are no other facilities, the organics become ours. It is OK to be realistic, but at the end of the day there may be no-one but us.' (Lester)

The nurses spoke of 'only having so many hours in the day', 'having to cut down the work rate', 'making sure they did not waste time because there were too many people to help', 'gauging their input', 'having to use the resources that we do have', being 'cost and time effective', and of 'it's all to do with economy of visiting'. The community psychiatric nurses clearly demonstrated that they were aware of 'juggling with resources', as can be seen in the following extracts:

> 'If a patient has local support, it helps us to decide the frequency of visits, the length of visits, how much input that person is going to need from us ... time is precious; it's all to do with economy, really.' (Adam)

> 'I only visit if I have something to offer. We don't visit psychogeriatrics on a regular basis. They are low priority. I'll do an assessment, maybe offer day care or support services, and we leave a card to say we have called. Unless we can offer a bed, we are just middle men for the consultant and get all the abuse. You can offer to put them on the waiting list but that is a lie − you can say it is for 3 months but you know it will be 3 years ...' (Kevin)

There were numerous examples given by the community psychiatric nurses which demonstrated how the availability or lack of resources shaped the possible scenarios of care between the community psychiatric nurses and the patients. The therapy was very subtly constructed according to, and being constrained by, the available resources rather than the patients' needs.

What resources were available to the nurses? There was some evidence that the community nurses developed their own new resources, especially group therapy situations; for example, a self-help group for lonely women with a history of mental illness was started by one nurse. There were other resources that were targeted as necessary developments, e.g. the creation of purpose-built day units, but the development of these was restricted by financial considerations. The nurses used other professionals as resources:

> 'I do like to refer on but that is not always possible, and you have to be realistic and take each case individually. That is another reason I see for working with social workers ... we cannot cope with all the problems and we should not try.' (Adam)

The facilities and resources in the two study areas differed (see chapter 3). Regardless of the details of actual resources, the nurses had to make decisions about who got what.

Fitting patients to resources Patients, despite the nurses' claims to provide care which catered for each individual, were not, in reality, offered 'individualised' care at all. They were 'fitted' to the available resources. As several of the community psychiatric nurses noted, it was easier for the nurses if they were able to gain information which they could then use:

'It's easier for both staff and patient if we can talk quite freely; the community psychiatric nurse can get to the root of the problem . . . he has more to work on.' (Eddie)

The nurses all had a clear idea of what help they could offer for specific problems: difficulties with money led to offers of help with budgeting; for problems of isolation and loneliness the offer of attendance at the day centre or at groups aimed at offering social stimulation were made; problems of low self-esteem and lack of confidence led to offers of group therapy; one-to-one therapy was offered for marital, family or relationship problems. As a nurse listened to a patient's description of difficulties, he would look for solutions to the problems from the stock of problems and related actions that the nurses carried around in their heads. This is similar to doctors' behaviour as described by Illsley (1980):

'Doctors spend many years acquiring a comprehensive compendium of knowledge about physiological, biochemical and psychological facts and events and a distinctive method of organizing that knowledge into states, processes and syndromes. At the end of their training they have learned how to obtain data from patients about their symptoms, to conduct physical examinations, to supplement the patient's report with other visible and tangible information and to request investigations about internal substances and processes invisible both to them and to the patient. They then organize the available data to correspond with learnt patterns signifying specific diseases and physiological processes. Their objective is also specific, *to link data patterns with acquired knowledge of causes and treatments.*' (my italics)

It is plausible to assume that the nurses acted in a similar way to doctors, because many of the community psychiatric nurses had had a hospital-based training influenced by the medical model.

Nurses talking to patients, therefore, had a dual purpose: in addition to facilitating the development of relationships with individual patients, referred to earlier, the information so gained helped to make extremely complicated situations and distress intelligible and manageable. Situations became manageable because the information given by the patient was 'fitted in' to a framework which the nurses had learned and could use.

The frameworks referred to by the nurses suggested that they used conceptual models of nursing (see chapter 2:2). Like doctors, the nurses made the patients' dialogue fit their knowledge base. Do the data suggest that community psychiatric nurses, like doctors, took a 'medical model' approach to patient care and fitted the patients' comments into a framework of physiological processes, causes and treatments of diseases? Some of the nurses did appear to use a 'medical model' framework in their practice, as evidenced by their comments that the aim of their discussions with patients was to 'get to the causes of, roots of or precipitants of illnesses'. There is also evidence from the data of the East Hospital nurses that much of the nurse activity was related to medication-giving and to actions relating to the monitoring of this treatment (in relation to the production of side-effects or symptom relief).

The 'medical model', however, was not used exclusively. The 'social model' of care was taken by some nurses who took a problem-solving approach to patients:

> 'It is my job to stop someone harming himself and improve his mental health. I want to get a comprehensive assessment to "treat" – I don't like the word "treat" – to help them look at a problem . . . if you use the word "treat" it is like you are going to cure them, but you are not, you are going in to help them.' (Jock)

A 'psychological model' was used by some nurses (see the example from Frank, p.143). The 'behavioural model' was also used, although minimally (see p.123). Individual nurses seemed to take an eclectic approach to the use of models, and one model was not used exclusively by one service.

The data suggest that the nurses controlled and manipulated conversations so that they were in a strong position of, in fact, not responding to expressed needs, but of responding to those which could be met by the available resources at the community psychiatric nurses' disposal. This point is illustrated in the excerpt below:

> 'Some folk don't like you prying into their personal lives. It takes longer to do an informal interview, in getting the information out, but I find it an awful lot better. I no longer do a formal interview . . . if I get my toes stood on, I just have to assess the situation and find out how they react to me. Some people just automatically blether and give away information that they think you want to know, others you've got to ask . . . I change my conversation and technique with the person and draw the information that is most relevant.' (Dick)

There were marked similarities in the thinking of the community psychiatric nurses as regards the 'fitting' of patients to the available treatment:

> 'If someone has been in hospital, they get out of the habit of talking to people, they feel different and don't want to join in normal social life. We'll get them to come to the group, otherwise all they do is sit in the home, do nothing and worry. We all do that. There is more time to think about how bad they feel. We want to try and stimulate them, to stop them brooding, becoming depressed. We don't want re-admission to hospital.' (Ivan)

There were also, however, some differences of opinion about 'fitting' patients to available treatment (see below).

Talking to patients appeared to be a reassuring activity in itself. This is graphically illustrated by the comments of one of the community psychiatric nurses:

'The more we know about patients, about how they react, the better control we have over situation and the less anxious we are about individuals.' (Graham)

It is also worth commenting that the talking/information-gathering may also have had the function of relieving the *client's* anxiety and distress through ventilation and sharing of feelings. This ventilation through discussion is referred to in the community psychiatric nurses' accounts, particularly in relation to crisis work, and is referred to in current literature (Oldfield, 1983). Furthermore, the nurses' conversations will also have had the effect of indicating to patients what to ask for, so, here again, we see how the nurses controlled the interactions with the patients/carers. Closer examination of the business of 'getting to know patients' revealed that 'developing relationships' was the nurses' shorthand for describing conversation which appeared free flowing, but in fact had the purpose of gaining particular information:

'. . . we actively encourage pill taking. The only way we can monitor this is by assessing their mental state: we talk to patients; we encourage them to talk about themselves. You can assess their mental state by talking to them. The patients themselves will tell us what we know all the time.' (Graham)

This was also the case when 'developing relationships' with the relatives. 'Getting to know the relatives' was useful to the nurses because, again, they may have found information which they could use. Some examples from the community psychiatric nurses serve to illustrate this process:

'Married people have, I feel, a lot more stress on them than single people, because of the stress of living with someone and the stress of children, perhaps; they have the stress of dealing with parents and in-laws; a lot will have money worries, sexual problems . . . if someone presents with a psychiatric disorder these are the most common reasons for frictions, this may be the reason that causes the illness. We'd want to try and change the way they functioned, the way they operated together; you can lower the level of anxiety, maybe relieve the psychiatric disorder. There may be non-therapeutic things going on in the family that would make your job difficult. So you'd want to know about them so that you could rectify any false views the patient has. Also, when you plan your programme, you'd plan it so that these people don't have access to intervention.' (Bert)

Developing relationships and getting to know patients served the purpose of acquiring information which allowed the nurses to fit patients and carers into available treatments. The nurses did not seem to be aware that they 'fitted' patients to treatment. This may well be because they strenuously attempted to keep faith with the ideology of 'individualised' care. The nurses, however, had a very real problem in maintaining an ideology of care focused on the individual, especially in the face of limited resources. Symptomatic of this difficulty, as demonstrated by the data, was that the community psychiatric nurses continually sought to legitimise their own actions and different ways of working.

Justifying the care
The notion of avoiding patient dependency The rationale of 'getting patients independent' fitted in with the philosophy of providing individualised care. The opposite notion, of 'avoiding getting patients dependent', was also used by the nurses. This not only fitted in with the ideology of 'individualised' care, but also allowed the nurses to withdraw services in a caring way and, in effect, helped the nurses to 'juggle resources'. This rationale was also used by the nurses to justify the care given.

Use of this rationale was vividly described in the following comments:

> 'You have to avoid setting up a dependency in people. You must look at that every few visits, right from the word go. Using contracts helps: I don't come over as "I'm going to cure you" but "I will help you. We will work together, and after so long, we will evaluate". It is including them and allowing them to take responsibility. Sometimes we have to bring the dependency thing out in the open.' (Lester)

This 'avoidance of dependency' rationale enabled the nurses, in a caring way, to withdraw services:

> 'Attendance at the day centre is gradually reduced, they are weaned off and their dependence lessened. We want to encourage them to be independent, and keep them at home, for the quality of life, for their own self-esteem. Nobody wants to attend the centre for a long time, and we encourage that. Another reason is to reduce the numbers of people attending and make room for others.' (Graham)

Patients' 'getting dependent' on the community nurses was seen predominantly as something to be avoided. One reason given was that a 'dependent patient' could not be weaned off treatment (the implication being that this person would be a long-term demand on resources). The logic of this stance would suggest that the nurses would be reluctant to offer prolonged care. The practice situation did not bear this out, the reality being that long-term care for patients was a feature of the work of community psychiatric nursing (see details of how the nurses described patients, p.139).

Some of the nurses described 'dependency' as 'becoming too emotionally attached' to the nurse; another reason given for 'avoiding dependency' was that if a patient became 'too attached' to (i.e. dependent on) any one nurse, it would make the nurse's successor's job difficult. This is an instance, again, of how present work is affected by consideration of (nursing) resources.

The reference to patients being 'over-involved' is interesting. The nursing literature on caring relationships warns against nurses becoming 'over-involved' with patients. It could be argued that if a *patient* is considered to be 'over-involved', this reflects badly on the nurse. Alternatively, the emphasis on avoiding dependency/ emotional attachment could arise out of the nurse's being unable to deal with the emotionally-charged nature of some nurse/patient relationships. In other words, the nurses dealt with the emotionally-charged relationship by curtailing it.

It could be argued that the nature of the 'caring relationship' places the patient in a 'dependent' relationship with the nurse (because of a requirement for help), and, hence, that dependency cannot be avoided. The nurses did not comment on dependency as being the result of the nurse/patient relationship and did not see this as a legitimate part of their work.

The nurses talked about 'promoting independence' and 'avoiding dependence' in tandem, but, clearly, this was a much more complex notion. The nurses did not speak openly of denying independence but, instead, referred to 'keeping a watchful eye' on some patients, 'providing limited support or contact' and 'providing constructive follow-up'. One of the services described 'on-call' patients who were unofficially 'kept on the books' because they were especially liked by particular nurses; these patients were not discharged. Denying independence was, therefore, considered legitimate in certain situations, usually in patients at risk of relapse.

Dependency was usually, but not always, considered to be a bad thing. Some of the nurses spoke of wanting to create a 'therapeutic dependency'. This described situations where the nurses considered long-term care or commitment (from the nurses) to be justifiable:

'You try and create a therapeutic dependency; so much attendance at a day centre, and we would make them do social skills, cooking, shopping . . . set out some sort of a programme so they would be able to talk about how they manage.' (Bert)

This description of care given mirrors that of the action involved in trying to 'promote independence'. The nurses tried to make patients independent by creating a 'therapeutic dependence', a link not focused on by the nurses themselves.

It was unclear from the data what criteria were used to determine the limits of therapeutic dependency, for example, when the dependency became 'untherapeutic'. There was some suggestion that, if the nurses felt they had nothing to offer, or if the patient was not progressing, changing or developing 'as expected' by the nurses, the dependency would be seen as untherapeutic and the nurse would take action to wean patients off treatment:

'I'd make out a programme and, if they did not work at it, I'd drop them a letter and say, "if you require further visits, please contact". I'll have called and they will not have stayed in, wasting everyone's time. There is no point. I'd tell them the reason why, that they are not willing; if they changed their mind, I'd try again.' (Ivan)

'Dependency' was also considered to be acceptable if this prevented a patient being admitted to hospital, as the following excerpt illustrates:

'There is nothing constructive about dependency unless it is in the psychotics; mostly it is a non-constructive thing. It is very difficult to get out of once you are into it, and it is not cost and time effective. Some people argue with this and say that if the community psychiatric nurse visiting keeps so-and-so out of hospital it is effective, and I can see that. But my view says something about my priorities, not necessarily about the service.'(Lester)

The nurses' reference to 'in the patient's interest'   The nurses referred to the actions they took as being 'in the patient's interest'; the benefits to patients, for example, of 'being independent', were frequently referred to by the nurses, e.g.:

'We want to instil in them a realistic sense of responsibility, not just socially but for themselves, allowing them the opportunity to be resourceful, so they feel better in themselves.' (Graham)

The nurses, continually argued that using the rationale of 'promoting independence' and 'avoiding dependence' was in the patient's interests (in the long term). This phrase, 'in the patient's interest', arising out of the ideology of 'individualised' care, could almost be described as a catchphrase which was used to legitimise whatever action the nurses wanted to do: any and all of the stances taken by the nurses were justified as being 'in the patient's interests'.

That the positions taken by the nurses were indeed 'in the patient's interests' is an assumption which can be challenged. Using the rationale of 'promoting independence' and 'avoiding dependence' clearly benefited the work of the nurses, helping them to structure and organise the work and to make demands more manageable. There were practical reasons for making a patient independent, for example, that the patients would no longer need the help of the community psychiatric nursing service. 'Denying independence' also had practical advantage, in that taking this stance allowed the nurses to cope and to avoid making unpleasant decisions, for example, discharging someone who might relapse. 'Avoiding dependence' allowed the nurses to reduce service provision and, in effect, share and stretch out the resources, while still maintaining a caring disposition.

The way in which the nurses worked was not just 'in the patient's interests' but also in the interest of 'other' patients. The data suggest that using the caring rationale served the interests of the nurses themselves and other patients and, overall, was in the interest of 'service provision'. By using this caring rationale, then, the nurses were in fact able, consciously or otherwise, to give an acceptable face to the lack of resources.

Some patients' interests were clearly not served by this approach: some were willing to be dependent on the nurses and they would have benefited from this had the nurses been obliging. This can be seen from the following account:

> 'I thought how sad it was, a young woman having to ask a visiting professional to walk her dog when she lived in a private housing estate with neighbours. The social worker did her a favour, not us ... there was an opportunity there to push her towards interacting with others that was lost ... it depends on the age, circumstances of the patient, everything comes into it ...' (Kevin)

This excerpt from the data shows that the dependency need of the patient was met by somebody else, in the above example a professional. This, in effect, meant that use of the 'getting independent' rationale resulted in what could be described as 'transferred dependency'. Patient dependence on the nurse was transferred to another professional.

Dependency could also be 'transferred' to the carers. This interpretation is supported by examination of the data on the occasions when the community psychiatric nurses talked about the relatives, carers or families. The nurses did try to share the dependency with the carers, as the following excerpts show:

> 'One patient is so demanding that the children are getting quite fed up ... we try and take some of that dependency off them, take some of the support for them, try and relieve them.' (Hamish)

> 'You would have a chat with the families and try and sort out the problem. And often having a chat about the patient, and getting out the anger towards a relative, is enough to maintain the situation for longer – it relieves the frustration and anxieties. It helps the family to know that somebody understands and cares, that they are not by themselves. If they are having difficulties, to talk about them and to know that somebody cares about their situation, this helps anyone.' (Colin)

It is unclear when it was considered legitimate to 'share the dependency'. It seemed far more likely that the nurses would 'transfer dependency' to the carers. The data in fact strongly suggest that 'patient interests' were maintained at the expense of the carers' interests as shown below.

The nurses' use of carers Scrutiny of the nurses' accounts suggest that the families were involved to help the nurses in the business of community psychiatric nursing. At the very least, families were involved in order that the community psychiatric nurses could obtain background information. As stated in the following extracts:

'If someone has family support you get a more objective picture of what is going on, a broader picture. Family are part of the information-gathering process.' (Frank)

'You see the relative to find out their side of the coin, to see how they find the patient ...' (Eddie)

This was particularly so for the families caring for patients suffering from dementia:

'If there is somebody there, there is always someone there to give a good record, an exact record of what has been happening between visits. It is a near-foolproof way to know if patients are taking the medication. We get a true history, if there have been any falls, sleepless nights ... Again you just want to establish what is going on – what in this case is appropriate to do. The more information you've got, the easier it is to decide what is the best thing to do for the patient.' (Dick)

Another reason for 'getting to know the relatives' was to 'check up' on the patient's story:

'Well, we see a patient, they say they are ill: we can find some biological symptoms, such as depression, there seems to be something there. But the patient doesn't always tell you everything that is going on in their life. A lot of people have court cases and, if you don't know any of the background information, you're going to say, "This person is unwell for no reason", treat them, give them a psychiatric label, when they are really responding to stress in their lives. It could be sorted out in other ways than psychiatric intervention.' (Bert)

This checking-up activity allowed the nurses to target treatment at the real problem (in the above case, the issues around the court appearance) rather than to treat an illness which might have been secondary (see chapter 2 and Caplan, 1964), and, further, was considered as crucial by the community psychiatric nurses in order to avoid giving someone a psychiatric label unnecessarily (see discussion below). Gaining information was also vital to the community psychiatric nurses for giving them feedback about treatment and progress:

'We try to keep a relationship going and develop a friendship with the family. They would be informed of progress or tell us if they see an improvement or deterioration.' (Hamish)

'Getting to know the patients and carers' was actually a fact-finding exercise which helped the community psychiatric nurses to determine care. It also became clear from the data that to know patients in their social context over a period of time was important. This was partly conveyed by the nurses' talking about 'developing relationships'. Use of the word 'developing' suggests movement over time, and the community psychiatric nurses made it clear that they did not get to know patients and carers in a series of individual and separate meetings. Rather, each meeting was interrelated with others, and the experience of the community psychiatric nurse in one situation predicted future action in another:

> 'If a patient is at loggerheads with the person with whom they live, the chances are that the community psychiatric nurse will get a lot of phone calls from the relatives complaining about the patient doing such-and-such. They'll complain of the slightest wee thing. I know they'll have had a fight or something the night before and I'll not race down: it'll have happened before; it's a case of making sure the relatives cannot manipulate you. With the folk that get on with the patient, you know they'd put up with an awful lot before they'd call: there must be something wrong and I'd visit straight away.' (Eddie)

The nurses, then, justified the care they gave by reference to information given by the relatives. Examination of the data revealed that 'getting to know the relatives' had a reassuring effect on the community psychiatric nurses:

> 'It makes us feel better, especially when they first come to the day centre, if we know they have someone to go home to. If something does crop up, the family will tell us and let us know.' (Graham)

The information gained from relatives and from involvement with the family was aimed at improving or maintaining the *patient's* health, not aimed at helping the carers. Much of the help that the relatives received, however, was coincidental. An excerpt from the interview data illustrates this point well:

> 'If the family has little contact with the patient, it would be quite useful to know why, and if, perhaps, there had been a family dispute or something like that, we may be able to find out exactly what had happened, smooth things over, get them communicating, which would alleviate the patient's isolation to a certain extent. There may have been problems in the family in relation to the dementia or paranoia, something like that – relatives may have found it difficult to cope with the patient, not really knowing what to do or what to say, because of the difference found in the elderly relative. We can discuss the problem with the family and explain the changes that are likely to occur and do occur with dementia and paranoia ... help them to try and understand why the elderly relative simply does not understand. It can help, in that it can cause a less strained relationship: the relatives can be more understanding of the problems and, therefore, have a better relationship with the patient; it is less of a strain on them ... it makes it easier for them to cope with the patients. It makes their coping ability greater.' (Colin)

'Supporting the relatives' has been stated in the literature as a reason for community psychiatric nursing development (see chapter 2); caring for the carers is, in theory, part of the ideology of community psychiatric nursing. The above excerpt shows that the community psychiatric nurses, when pushed to explain why they are interested in specific information, appear concerned for the carer. The data also suggest, however, that this is of interest only inasmuch as it affects the care given to patients. The nurses were not interested in helping the carer to cope *unless this in turn was beneficial to the patient, or to the nurse's management of the patient.* Carers, it seems, were not helped in their own right.

Taken further, the interview data suggest that the nurses seemed to use the availability of carers to assist in making the community psychiatric service work. This is most obvious in the above exerpt, where the explicit aim of the work of the community psychiatric nurse was to 'increase the coping capacity' of the carer; this, of course, in turn had the effect of enabling the patient to remain in the home situation.

Care which the community psychiatric nurses could give to the carers was limited by two factors. First, it was limited by the abilities of the community psychiatric nurses to develop relationships with the carers:

'It depends on personalities: I may not be able to communicate too well with some families, but with others someone else could.' (Colin)

Second, it was constrained by the availability of resources to the community psychiatric nurses:

'Some families struggle on and it's not until we are called in that we can put support in . . . I assess the situation and try and say to them, "I can understand why you want to look after your wife; if you got a home help in to do the heavy work, that would give you more time to look after her" . . . some families will go round and make mum's lunch or whatever. If they are happy with that, fine, but it can become a bit of a burden, so I would suggest meals-on-wheels . . . aids can be given, it all boils down to the fact that everything I've said is to make life easier for the person who cares. Sometimes it isn't possible to relieve the situation. A lot of the time you can't.' (Dick)

The data showed that the community nurses were concerned for the carers, but limited resources (including psychiatric nursing manpower) restricted the help which could be offered to carers.

'You always try and involve families, but this would involve a considerably larger amount of work if you wanted to involve the families in a constructive way. The family may not necessarily be part of the illness, but with families with any pathology, we're treating a sick relationship not a sick individual. Most families have some pathology, they don't know that is happening, don't know what to do for the best, don't want to push too hard. That sort of situation is quite easy to deal with, but I'm talking about families that are resistive to the suggestions of the community psychiatric nurse. If the family is involved with the patient's illness, the patient will not get better and stay better, if it is the family dynamics that are sick. So we are looking for a compromise,

modifying family attitudes so that the patient's illness can be looked after
... to help the patient reach his optimum level of functioning. That is not
necessarily my idea of "better", it is to do with the patient's idea of where
he is going and how he is functioning.' (Jock)

Here again, we see how the work of the community psychiatric
nurses was influenced by resources and how the community psychiatric nurses 'juggled resources' to make the service work. The carers
were not just sources of information but were used by the community
psychiatric nurses to help to plan the community psychiatric nursing
input:

'Knowing the support system affects our input, helps plan our involvement. We find out what goes on, and decide our approach, what to use,
what to encourage ... time spent with one person could be cut down if
we know there are people around that do certain things.' (Adam)

'For one you know how much support you need to give – go in every day
or whether you can share with a caring relative.' (Bert)

This aspect of community provision of nursing care was in some
ways quite unexpected. The literature suggested that informal carers,
most often female kin, would be involved in care of the mentally ill in
the home situation. That the community psychiatric nurses used the
availability of carers to gauge the level of nursing input is an
indication of how pressed the nurses were.

This is quite different from the role of relatives in relation to nursing
in the hospital situation. Regardless of the availability of relatives, the
nursing establishment of wards is estimated on the number and
condition of patients. Involvement of relatives in hospital wards is
encouraged or discouraged according to local management
preferences; carer involvement in day-to-day care is not expected. If
it was, it would doubtless raise questions about manpower
deficiencies and about whether relatives would then be expected to
do more, and for more patients. Debates about the role of volunteers
and workers on job-creation schemes in the hospital situation are
evident in the contemporary nursing press (Kratz, 1987). The current
shortage of trained staff (see chapter 1) and the proposal that future
nurse learners be taught outside the hospital situation (United
Kingdom Central Council, 1985) may mean that the role of carers in
hospital will be prominent in future.

This brief excursion into the role of relatives in hospitals illustrates
the different expectation of caring relatives when compared to the
community setting. What has been, or is, responsible for these
differences? What were the expectations of the community
psychiatric nurses with regard to family involvement, and what
limited these? These questions were not explored in depth, but they
remain areas worthy of further investigation.

There was some evidence from the data that the community

psychiatric nurses were unsure of how much to get involved with carers. The following was said by one nurse:

'It is my job to be aware of the mental health of the family, but I get involved to varying degrees. It depends who else is involved. I'm not sure how much we should get involved but what happens is that you don't usually have a lot of choice. We can't draw the boundaries.' (Lester)

The nurses seemed to be in a 'catch 22' situation, where concern for the patient, learned during training, was reinforced by the existence and perpetuation of resources which catered for patients. This focus on individualised (patient) care compounded the lack of interest in or ability of the nurses to care for the carers, and conflicted with the expressed wishes of the nurses 'to help the carers'. What resulted was that the nurses provided as much care as they could to the carers (by listening and being available) and, for the most part, enabled carers to continue in their caring role. The nurses' work with the carers appeared more to do with 'juggling resources' and making the system work than with helping the carers.

It will be remembered that the nurses, by 'showing that they cared', were able to 'manage crises', 'provide early treatment' and 'prevent admissions to hospital'. All three approaches were justified by the nurses because the patients could then remain at home, which was considered preferable to institutional care. Hospital was considered by the nurses to be a resource which was only used as a last resort, and 'avoiding blocking beds' was a justification for keeping patients in their own homes for as long as possible. The families' ability and capacity to continue caring for a mentally-ill relative also influenced the nurses' decision to admit patients to hospital, and the nurses stated that they would not 'prevent admission to hosptial *at all costs*'. It was unclear what 'costs' were targeted as being an indication of the limits to the provision of care at home by the carers. Taking an approach of 'showing that they cared', however, detracted from the reality of service provision, which was that limited resources were available. It could be argued, for instance, that 'lack of resources' and inability to provide optimum care could produce 'crisis'.

Labelling Another effect of using the notions of 'promoting independence' and 'avoiding dependence' was that this had ramificiations in the way that community psychiatric nurses described patients. Some comments of the community psychiatric nurses suggested that they wished to avoid 'labelling' patients. Avoiding labelling was specifically discussed by the nurses, as the following excerpt shows:

'Once you've labelled someone as psychiatrically ill, it becomes an illness in itself. People look upon them as being ill and it is hard to get rid of that label, whether the person has had any psychiatric illness or not. They are looked upon as a deviant in society, as being less than normal, as being socially inadequate.' (Bert)

The evidence below suggests that the nurses, paradoxically, did indeed 'label' patients. One cannot help but ask why the nurses did this, what purpose the labels had, and, similarly, what effect the labelling had. These issues are explored below.

'Labelling' describes the use of short, descriptive tags which define individuals rather than objectively describing their behaviour, and which exert an effect on the individual's subsequent career. Labelling theorists argue that the most crucial step in the development of deviant behaviours is the experience of being publicly labelled 'deviant'. Whether or not this happens depends 'not so much on what he does as on what others do' (Becker, 1963).

Goffman (1961, 1963, 1964) and Scheff (1966) describe certain stages involved in the labelling process in relation to mental illness. Diagnoses are examples of such labels:

'Putting a label on a patient can invalidate the patient – "you are invalid, and what you say is therefore invalid. You are sick because your label says so". Diagnosis can therefore become a way of restraining people and of rendering them even more impotent than they were when they started. To say someone is neurotic, psychotic or psychopathic or schizophrenic is not just a scientific statement. It can become a way of making a value judgement about the patient and putting him down.' (Mitchell, 1973)

Patients are not only labelled on admission to hospital; there is evidence to suggest that patients can also be labelled in the community by professionals (Penfold and Walker, 1983), and by society (Mechanic, 1968; Page, 1984).

Rosenhan (1973) has shown how normal people can be labelled 'schizophrenic' and how normal behaviour can then be misinterpreted or overlooked. Kreitman (1961) conducted a study where pairs of psychiatrists independently interviewed 90 outpatients; they found that there was only a 50% chance of agreement on symptoms and diagnosis. Other authors have also commented on the unreliability of psychiatric diagnosis (Bannister et al, 1964; Kendell, 1975). More recent work sponsored by the World Health Organisation has shown that the reliability of psychiatric diagnosis can be improved through the use of agreed definition of terms (World Health Organisation, 1978). The application of psychiatric diagnostic 'labels', despite their imprecision, is liable to have relatively powerful effects. (This fact was acknowledged in the present study, as demonstrated by the comments of Bert, above.)

Rosenthal and Fode (1963) observed a strong association between 'problem' patients and the failure to establish an organic basis to the illness. Jeffery (1979) suggests that, for his casualty doctors, the terms 'problem patient' and 'psychiatric patient' were virtually synonymous.

These findings are similar to those of Becker (1963), Strong (1980) and Hughes (1981). There is research evidence to suggest, then, that doctors label patients. Research has also demonstrated that nurses use labels in their work with patients. Stockwell (1972) showed that, on general wards, nurses identify popular and unpopular patients; nurse/patient interaction was found to be related to this perception and psychiatric patients were overtly rejected or ridiculed. May and Kelly (1982) suggested that psychiatric nurses perceive patients as either 'chancers, pests or poor wee souls', each category legitimising a particular nurse interaction. These authors noted that:

> 'Problem or disliked patients are those who call attention to the fragility of nursing authority by rejecting, implicitly or explicitly, the services – help, advice, treatment – that the psychiatric nurse stands ready to provide.'

In view of the above comments, and the fact that most community psychiatric nurses do not receive post-registration training (see chapter 2), it is reasonable to assume that community psychiatric nurses continue practices learned in the institutional setting. The evidence from the interview data clearly demonstrated that community psychiatric nurses do 'label' patients.

The nurses' use of labels Getting to know the patient and carers over a period of time had a strong influence on the work of the community psychiatric nurses, and resulted in the nurses describing patients in terms of the length of contact with the community psychiatric nursing service. Descriptions of patients with lengthy contact with the psychiatric services included 'chronic', 'long term', 'old', 'known', 'regulars', 'having a long history or lengthy experience of psychiatric care' or a 'psychiatric background', 'been on the books for years' and 'professional patients'. In contrast, there were patients described as 'acute', 'short term', 'recent contacts', 'unknowns' or 'an unknown quantity', and 'new referrals'. Visits to new patients were described as 'cold visits', 'first visits' and 'initial assessments'. The influence these descriptions had on the community psychiatric nurses' work is demonstrated in the following excerpt:

> 'When notes are available, if someone has a history you use that for guidance. I'm less professional with the psychotics. You fall into the role of familiarity. That is a particular danger with depot drugs – you give them the injection and maybe don't look so closely at them ... with first referrals, you go into the house from scratch and spend a lot of time on that person.' (Kevin)

Work with new patients was more anxiety provoking for the community psychiatric nurses, and there was no information initially on which they could work. This anxiety may be related to the fact that the nurses had not yet legitimised their approach to patients. As the above excerpt indicates, work with a 'known' patient had its problems too.

The following excerpt demonstrates the linkage of 'new' and 'old' patients with the notions of crisis work and avoidance of care in hospital.

> 'There are people who have been on the psychiatric roundabout, who have been seen by psychiatric doctors and have adopted the sick role. Those not diagnosed as psychiatrically ill are easier to work with; it's easier for them to accept that they have a problem. Most of them are frightened of being diagnosed as mentally ill; things are more acute, the pain is still there. With those who have been diagnosed, etcetera, added on to that there is sometimes the idea of, "I must go into hospital to be made better"; with them it is more difficult to prevent hospitalisation and work with problems.' (Lester)

A 'management of crisis' approach (see chapter 2) tended to be taken with 'new' referrals and also with 'old' patients for whom hospital care had been unsuccessful. This can be seen from the following example:

> '... you do a little bit of digging about ... it becomes apparent that all these people need is some outside intervention to help them through the stressful period, then usually you don't see them again. A great deal of psychiatry seems to be a bit of that now, especially the new referrals – a lot of new referrals, you'll see them once and they are not really a psychiatric case but there is something needing ... it is useful to know that for the next time something happens ... it is a good learning situation. When we know the patient, we don't see the situation as a new crisis but as a pattern to the patient's life, they become ill in a certain way. If a patient is running about hallucinating, you would think that this person should be in hospital, but from experience we know that this person is a gross hysteric. You could go out and give them some tranquillisers to calm them down. If you take them into hospital, you are uprooting them from their families. You are disrupting all the supportive services that are there – it is better to go and do something at home.' (Bert)

Other researchers have found that the work of community psychiatric nurses varies depending on the length of patient contact. Sladden (1979), for instance, found (based on the nurses' inter-pretations of their contacts) that activities aimed at changing patients' behaviour directly (using advice, persuasion, or warnings), or indirectly (using a cognitive approach aimed at developing insight and understanding), were more frequently used at initial contacts and, in particular, where community psychiatric nurses had noticed deterioration. It was surprising that the community psychiatric nurses' activities were significantly related to initial contacts, as one would have expected these activities to be related to the community psychiatric nurses' longer-term work (with both patients and families).

The East and West Hospital nurses used other descriptions and labels. The patients were judged by the community psychiatric nurses in relation to past responses to treatment, and were described accordingly. 'Dependent patients' were referred to by the community psychiatric nurses and described as 'a drain on resources', 'a draw on the helping agencies', 'demanding', 'psychopathic manipulators', 'getting secondary gain out of the sick role', 'attention seekers', and 'professional patients'. The community psychiatric nurses had individual lexicons – a favourite range of descriptions for patients who did not 'fit in' to, and co-operate with, the treatment offered. There was a common understanding as to the meaning of these lexicons, even across the two community psychiatric nursing services studied. Patients that did not 'fit in' to the available resources were variously described by the community psychiatric nurses as 'unresponsive', 'difficult', 'irregular attenders', 'defaulters', 'resistant to therapy', 'unmotivated', 'lacking insight' or 'manipulators'. No mention was ever made by the nurses themselves about the deficiencies of the community psychiatric nursing services offered.

These labels were used by the nurses to describe patients whom they found difficult to help, in other words who were unable to be made 'independent'. There was an abundance of 'negative' descriptions (perhaps, logically, because those who would qualify for the positive range of descriptions are, by implication, no longer in need of help, i.e. they are independent and, therefore, ready for discharge). These labels served the purpose of helping the nurses to cope with failures, patients who failed to become independent and patients who failed to fit into the available services and resources. The labels were used by the nurses to legitimise the work, and helped the nurses to decide who got what treatment. Furthermore, the use of labels also helped the nurses to cope, first, with patients who did not fit into treatment, and second, with managing the nursing service. So, here again, we see the importance of 'justifying the care' and 'juggling resources'.

The labels were meant for 'in-house' use; this was made quite clear to me because I was treated as 'in-house'. In both research areas, I was made to feel welcome because of my practical experience as a community psychiatric nurse; there was a feeling of camaraderie during the interview sessions and some of the nurses joked in a conspiratorial manner about the 'labels' they used. This, combined with the comments of the nurses, suggested that the 'labels' were for the private use of the community psychiatric nurses. The data in fact suggest further that use of 'labels' facilitated communication between the nurses. This is demonstrated clearly in the following excerpt:

'I don't go in with the idea that someone is chronic, I go in to help that person as much as I can. It is a term I would use with you, not with them. I don't really even look on them as chronic, they are a person to me. It's just a piece of shorthand to describe what they are like ...' (Ivan)

The above comments suggest that the nurses did not intend to harm the patients. Taking note of the above theory of labelling, however, there are implications in describing patients as 'dependent' (or whatever), and this 'labelling' may have adverse effects on the patients. The theory suggests that the nurses' use of negative labels to describe the patients will result in the patients being viewed in terms of these 'labels'. This could have several undesirable effects:

- patient improvement and changes for the better may not be observed by the nurses (who may pay more attention to aspects of behaviour which necessitate the use of the 'dependent' label);
- other professionals will pick up these labels and perceive the patients negatively, as difficult and demanding, for instance;
- patients, themselves, may also begin to accept the labels and believe that they are in need, dependent, demanding, a drain on resources, etc., and begin to conform to these descriptions (an effect which works against the thrust of the nurses' therapy, which is to help individuals to be autonomous, self-sufficient and independent).

This aspect of the nurses' work could mean that, for some patients, the nurses may be inadvertently perpetuating patient dependency.

The nurses' view of patients   The nurses' use of labels is more than a mechanism of communication. The labels demonstrate how the nurses viewed patients. The interview findings show that individual prejudices or preconceptions may affect the work of community psychiatric nurses. This is contrary to what might be expected of nursing work, where an assumption of the nurse/patient relationship is that the nurse should adopt an 'objective and impartial' attitude (see chapter 2).

As discussed above, several authors have noted that psychiatric nurses can have prejudiced views of patients which can, in turn, determine treatment. The following example shows this process is evident in the work of the community psychiatric nurses:

> 'It depends on the condition of the patient as well. I know someone who we would have had no difficulty going shopping with or getting her chocolate because she was a pet patient and she also had a terminal illness. That changes how you behave; there is someone else, youngish, just neurotic, who wanted us to do things like walk the b... dog ...'(Kevin)

In this excerpt from the data, the terminally-ill patient was seen as a 'poor wee soul', and the other, as a 'chancer' (see above comments and May and Kelly, 1982). The second patient was described as 'neurotic'. McIlwaine (1980) demonstrated that neurotic patients are viewed negatively by psychiatric nurses (in the hospital situation). The data here suggest that only some of the community psychiatric nurses held these negative opinions of 'neurotic' patients; an extract from the data illustrates this:

'Neurotics and hysterics tend to act how they feel ... you know they're not acting in a bizarre way, it's not because they are mad. It's because they are distressed about something and you want to push them to look at it ... you want to relieve the distress ... reflect back on them what they are doing and at the same time reassure them, saying that how they feel is a more effective way of getting what they want and if they do this it won't be the end of the world.' (Frank)

The example shows that this nurse, far from being negative, was prepared to take a constructive approach to management of the neurotic patients in his care. The data show overwhelmingly, however, that how the nurses viewed and described patients affected their work. The nurses were aware that their views of patients might be judgmental. This was most obvious during some of the interviews when the nurses stopped describing their work and commented that they treated all the patients 'just the same'. This was clearly contradicted by elaboration of different types of treatment being offered to different patients, as shown in the following excerpt:

'We would offer the same sort of thing for someone who was isolated and for someone with family support. But you tend to be more aware of just how they are managing and ask more about how they are coping. With a family around patients will be attended to ... but really we do try to treat everyone the same.' (Colin)

An explanation of this reaction may be that the nurses felt discomfort at the realisation that they carried out 'patient triage' in relation to offering treatment. The exercise of discretion is considered to be one of the prime attributes of professional work, but it may be that the nurses found it difficult to acknowledge the extent to which they sorted patients and decided who should be given what resources.

At times, the nurses acknowledged the influence of their personal judgments and stated that their opinion might be wrong. Nevertheless, the judgments did affect the way the nurses managed patients, as is shown in the following excerpt:

'I'm thinking of neurotic hysterics who would go to a GP and, for the sake of peace and quiet and tranquillity, to keep cases at bay, he'll put people on anxiolytics or sleeping tablets when they really shouldn't be. The GPs are putting them on it because the patient demands it, not because the patient really needs it. That is a very subjective thing. It is my opinion that they shouldn't be on it. If I feel someone is on medication and doesn't need it, I would be looking closely at his symptoms and getting a mental approach to his symptoms. . . Trying to deal with their feelings instead of hiding behind valium, with the ultimate objective of getting them off it, not taking it away from them, but getting them to see that they don't need it; let them see that they can manage without it . . . because you can't hide behind valium for years. You're just putting off the evil hour.

'The GP is treating symptoms, not treating the person as someone with problems. He is treating the objective complaint without looking at why, without looking at why they feel tense. Part of our remit is to look at why people feel tense, not just pour valium down their throats . . . some patients need a prop and can only deal with their feelings if they have medication. It is very much an emotive subject.

'We're talking about my opinion. I'm not sure whether my opinion should come into it, but it is very difficult to keep your opinions and feelings out of it . . . we want to get away from producing chronic invalids who've been on valium for years and this is compounded by their unresolved feelings, and they are addicted to the stuff . . .' (Frank)

This excerpt from the data clearly shows how the nurse's judgments determined treatment and provided a rationale for his management of patients. It is obvious, too, that concern for the patient is central in this account.

The fact that the community psychiatric nurses hold prejudiced views of patients and carers is not necessarily bad. Hume and Pullen (1986) consider that the varied opinions of psychiatric nurses about patients are an important facet of treatment in the multidisciplinary setting. Burgess (1981) talks of the concept of 'stalls', including 'judgmental feelings', which are unavoidable factors that impede the therapeutic process. Peplau (1952) emphasises the importance of the nurse assessing his own interpersonal behaviour as it affects the therapeutic relationship, the work roles of the psychiatric nurse and the phases of the nurse/patient relationship. There are also particular difficulties for psychiatry, and, hence, in the work of community psychiatric nurses in particular, in maintaining a balance between subjective perception and objective data in psychiatric practice.

The work of psychiatry has less scientific rigour to control its practice than has traditional medical practice. The seminal work of Zola (1972) and Illich (1976), and others since, e.g. Illsley (1980), have clearly argued that medicine is a 'system of social control':

'The uncomfortable suspicion has been frequently voiced that some forms of medical diagnosis and labelling, particularly those relating to mental illness or insanity, are convenient means of locking away individuals whose behaviour is uncomfortable for society. Psychiatrists themselves are concerned about its uses in the USSR as a means of silencing political critics. The situation is exacerbated by the fact that decision-rules for the diagnosis of illness are not so strict as those for determining criminal behaviour; nor are they so open to public view and judgment. It does not, however, require such extreme cases to make the point that the more medicine moves from technological intervention in organic conditions to the surveillance and modification of everyday behaviour, the more likely it is that it will be involved in controversial issues on which its motivation and authority can be challenged. This is an uncomfortable position for a profession which has based its claim to status and autonomy on scientific principles, and which has emphasised its freedom from political and social values.' (Illsley, 1980)

The community psychiatric nurses in the study were clearly aware of their role in this 'system of social control', as shown below:

'Some of the work is to do with getting people adjusted to retirement ... getting them advice; there are pamphlets you can pick up ... getting voluntary workers to pop in, or getting them involved in the Church. I want to improve their quality of life, improve their outlook, get them accepted ...' (Jock)

We have seen, so far, that the community psychiatric nurses made decisions about who should receive what care, and that they used various devices to justify the care, such as using the avoidance of dependency rationale and referring to the work as being 'in the patient's interest'. The nurses also legitimised the work by using labels. Another way in which the nurses endorsed their practice was by seeking legitimacy from the group: they justified their less than impartial attitude by seeking group consensus and approval at meetings of their peers.

The nurses' use of group consensus The community psychiatric nurses talked about 'playing it safe'. This was, in effect, a phrase which described a range of activities in which the nurses engaged, which put limits and checks on their behaviour. One way of 'playing it safe' was that the nurses did not exclusively rely on their own judgment: 'second opinions' were sought. These sometimes involved the family:

'You speak to the family to substantiate what the other person is telling you. You get another view: if someone has been married for ages, you've got to admit that that person knows more about the patient than you do, and can see changes that you are unlikely to pick up and miss.' (Adam)

'Pooling opinions' and coming to a decision based on the weight of opinion was another way in which the community psychiatric nurses made difficult decisions and discussed approaches to patient care:

'You see the relative to find out their side of the coin, to see how they find the patient, so I can compare what I think and what the GP thinks to what the relatives and the patient are saying.' (Eddie)

The opinions of the patients, families and other professionals were pooled. Multidisciplinary meetings also took place in the parent hospitals (more so in East Hospital) and these afforded opportunity to discuss patient management and approaches. Case conferences were also held if a situation was particularly problematic. Both community psychiatric nursing services had regular community psychiatric nursing meetings where opinions could be pooled and ideas shared:

> 'Sometimes you find yourself a wee bit insecure in that you wonder if somebody could make trouble for you. I would discuss that with my colleagues and ask them what they thought. Provided everyone agreed, I would stick with my decision and then speak to the consultant.' (Kevin)

The community psychiatric nurses had to make complicated and difficult decisions about patient management. The nurses were aware of the possibility of things going wrong, and talked of creating 'safety nets', which was how the nurses referred to the letters written to GPs if a patient was discharged. These always offered the possibility of re-referral and future treatment:

> 'We find that the ones that attend irregularly are not motivated to get help. If it's just a case of not being motivated, then there's no point in pushing them; you'd probably wait for another crisis and pick them up again. But you would inform the GP, keep everyone in the picture – we'd be willing to take them on again.' (Hamish)

The nurses also talked about having 'contingency plans'. Often the nurses had alternative treatment plans which could be implemented if the first approach to care failed. In East Hospital, these were sometimes formally written down in an 'at risk' register in the admission ward (see p.150). It is unclear at what stage of therapy this was undertaken, but the name suggests that this was used when nurses were anxious about patients' welfare.

There were instances cited in the data where nurses were challenged about their treatment decisions and actions (by relatives, by other professionals and by lay people in the community). This resulted in the nurses having joint meetings to compare the opinions of colleagues, and this often resulted in discussions with the consultant. There was evidence, therefore, that the service closed ranks to support the nurses' exercise of professional discretion.

My impression, based on limited attendance at staff meetings, was that the aim of multidisciplinary meetings was formally to review progress and to make decisions about patient care; the feelings of the nursing staff about patient management were rarely explored. An additional impression gained of these meetings (and based on the comments of the nurses) was that the organisation of the nursing services, particularly in East Hospital, was influenced by other professions, especially medicine.

What Gouldner (1959) has called 'latent social identities' may be evident in the work of the community psychiatric nurses. These are identities which are not culturally prescribed as relevant to or within rational organisations, and which intrude upon and influence behaviour in interesting ways. This is an area of study worthy of future investigation and separate detailed examination.

The nurses' work and the bureaucracy The varied ways in which the nurses handled similar situations and the fact that the nurses' attitudes influence practice leads one to ask how far the individual nurses let their personal feelings intrude on their work, and to what extent the bureaucracy limited individual work practices.

The data suggest that there was a certain amount of bureaucratic control over the community psychiatric nurses, which maintained a check on the individual scope of the work. The nurses felt that their work was being monitored, as shown by the following comments:

> 'It [the work] is up to you. You don't get that many wasted visits anyway. If it went up to 50% "they" might be a wee bit wary. It is quite in order if you work that way. We keep a "Kalamazoo", the record that the district nurses use.' (Kevin)

This nurse, then, talking about his individual work pattern, the irregular nature of which incurred 'wasted visits', inferred that 'they', i.e. the organisation, would inform him if this was unacceptable practice. This assumption was based on the fact that individual community nurses were obliged to complete detailed day-to-day records of their work practices (statistical returns, Kardexes or Kalamazoos). The controls exerted by the bureaucracy were few, and these measures, with their quantitative focus (McKendrick, 1981a,b) did little to examine performance on a qualitative level.

The nurses, themselves, put checks and limits on their activities by working within self-made guidelines. Care was also legitimised by the use of agreed policies (see p.150). The use of these policies and planned inputs portrayed the image of the nurse as 'being organised'. It will be remembered that no formal assessment tools (Barker, 1986) were described or referred to by the community nurses (see p.123). In the absence of undertaking 'systematic assessments', or using measuring tools to assess input and measure output, it could be argued that 'being organised' was a facade used by the community psychiatric nurses which obscured the reality of the effect of the community psychiatric nurses' attitudes and which, in turn, may have served the purpose of offering some legitimacy to the work.

Murray (1974) has stated that the nurse alone is unable to assess the effects of attitudes and feelings. He commented:

> 'Therapeutic treatment of patients is not something that can be left to the good will of the staff. Procedures should be devised which will help the staff deal with the stress and frustrations that arise in the mental hospital setting. Mental health professionals should regularly evaluate their attitudes and responses to patients. They should also attempt to examine objectively the social system in which they work to discover the effects of the system's internal operations on the patient's behaviour and its

effects on their own behaviour. In addition, they should examine their role in the behaviours that patients demonstrate ...'

Although Murray is talking about hospital-based nurses, the issues raised are equally pertinent to the community psychiatric nurses, and suggest that regular forums should be available, where patient management and the nurses' feelings are discussed.

Menzies (1960) has shown that general nursing is organised to contain the anxiety of staff. One cannot help but wonder how far the community psychiatric nursing work patterns evolved to cope with the anxiety aroused from developing new and autonomous work patterns and from juggling resources. Previous studies focusing on community psychiatric nursing suggest that some of the activities and responses of the community psychiatric nurses could be to anxiety, rather than to a systematic assessment of need (Hunter, 1978; Sladden, 1979).

Hunter and Sladden studied the work of psychiatric nurses in community settings. The increased admission rate found in Hunter's study could be the community psychiatric nursing response to coping with anxiety. Sladden found that a decreased frequency of visits followed detection of deterioration. It is possible that this response could be to anxiety rather than to systematic assessment of the need for visits. Sladden also found that community psychiatric nurses 'held on to' patients. It could be argued that this finding is symptomatic of community psychiatric nurse anxiety surrounding case-load management.

There is evidence of anxiety in the present accounts given by the nurses about their work; 'getting to know the patients and relatives' was partly undertaken because of this. The introduction of 'supervision' (see chapter 5) into the work of the community psychiatric nurses may be a helpful strategy which could provide some support for the nurses. In the present study, existing meetings of the community psychiatric nurses were used to discuss business and administrative matters. Patient management was discussed regularly on an informal basis by the nurses themselves, and was most evident during a 'crisis' when urgent decisions needed to be made. 'Supervision' sessions (Community Psychiatric Nurses Association, 1985), which allow the nurses the opportunity to focus on attitudes and feelings about management, and afford opportunity for insightful practice or staff development, were lacking. The managers of the services are in an ideal position to introduce an element of supervision into the practice of the community psychiatric nurses.

The findings in this study demonstrate that decisions on which patients receive care are made by the individual community psychiatric nurses. Kalkman (1974) says that nurses are not independent practitioners as they depend on doctors' referrals and prescriptions of patient care. The CPNA Survey (Community Psychiatric Nurses Association, 1985b), however, suggests that community psychiatric nurses receive only 82% of their referrals from GPs or psychiatrists; referrals are also taken from district nurses, health visitors, social services and directly from patients and relatives. This could indicate that community psychiatric nurses are moving towards being autonomous practitioners.

This move seems to be reflected in debate within community psychiatric nursing (Community Psychiatric Nurses Association, 1985c), and in nursing generally, (Royal College of Nursing, 1981) and suggests that this is an issue of concern. Clearly, if the work of the community psychiatric nurse is broadened to include early detection of mental distress, issues of accountability, responsibility and autonomy will increase. The West Hospital community psychiatric nurses operated an open referral system (see chapter 3) and the data suggest that individuals developed their own working practices. In this sense, the community psychiatric nurses are operating autonomously and with very few controls. The checks and safeguards described by the community nurses, which they imposed on their work, are a way in which the nurses have evolved practice to preserve some sense of accountability and responsibility.

The nurses' use of moral considerations   There are moral aspects in the business of 'juggling resources' and 'justifying care', and the community psychiatric nurses relied on moral considerations to legitimise their work. Similarly, bureaucratically-driven decisions, influenced by resources in themselves, presented as moral decisions. These moral considerations, which significantly influenced the nursing practices, are presented.

'Moral responsibility' is referred to by Rhodes (1986) as 'consideration of one's obligations to act for the overall good of others and society'. The nurses seemed to consider it preferable to help as many patients as possible. This was the rationale behind group work: 'You can deal with eight or nine folk in an afternoon in a group. There is no way you could deal with that on your own' (Ivan).

This choice, to help many rather than few, can be traced partly to the current emphasis in practice on 'efficiency' arising from central government's stress, since the early 1980s, on efficiency savings and the implementation of the Griffiths Management Stucture (Department of Health and Social Security, 1983). The importance that managers place on quantitative statistics (see p.56) to evaluate community psychiatric nursing activities serves to combine with this to make the choice of treating many patients preferable to that of treating few.

To pursue a policy of maximising benefit to the community at large, however, it may be necessary to ignore the plight of others who may be expensive as regards resource use. Taken to the extreme, this argument suggests that some individuals are expendable for the sake of the good of others. There is, in fact, some evidence of the nurses taking this stance, as the following comments show: 'We don't visit psychogeriatrics on a regular basis, they are low priority' (Kevin). This is a dimension of psychiatric work that is not as relevant for psychiatric nurses working in wards. Here, demands for care are controlled by hospital or admission policies and are limited by the work of others in the team. The solitary nature of the work and the variety of contacts in the community setting may mean that the community psychiatric nurses have to decide how to limit the demands made of them.

There are alternative options open to community psychiatric nurses. One alternative, discussed by Downie and Telfer (1980) is the notion of 'equal consideration', which is demand for *consistent* treatment between individuals and the use of a rule which can be formulated as a guideline to practice. This demand for consistency clashes with the personalised nature of the caring relationship which stresses the individuality of situations. Nevertheless, there was evidence that the nurses used and applied some rules consistently. These rules, called 'policies', resulted from the community psychiatric nurses, as a group, agreeing to take a common approach to situations, as can be seen from the following excerpt:

> 'If someone has had past suicide attempts and you thought that they were really ill, depressed and didn't want to come into hospital, you would think twice about leaving a person out and treating them in the community; in that case you would maybe think about whether they were certifiable – should they be in hospital and in care?
> 'If the past suicide attempt had been psychopathic-type manipulation behaviour, you have to find out what the *policy* was and what the last letter said, if this person had to be treated again or what. Are they to be given drugs? It all depends on what the *policy* is . . .
> 'The person may have presented with what seemed to be a psychiatric disorder, but on investigation it turns out to be a reaction to stress in their lives. People have said, "They are psychopathic, but let's see if we can help them, let's do A, B and C"; and every time you do this, and they wouldn't do anything, you would say, "There is not much more we can do for you. We will set up this network so that, if it happens again, we'll come and see you, and if things have changed we'll try and help you."
> 'In our crisis list there are people at risk, but there are also information sheets for patients who are not to be admitted in any circumstances. But it is not quite like that; there is a little bit of information, and we would go and assess the situation and if things have changed, we can form a new treatment plan.' (Bert)

Agreed policies seemed to give legitimacy to care provision. Consistency is necessary if care is seen to be fair, but this is not a sufficient condition for 'fairness': a consistently-applied rule, for example, that all schizophrenic patients be refused hospital admission could still be thought of as unfair.

The provision of *equality* of treatment may be an option, but this is not realistic as it would be unreasonable to spend the same amount of time and money regardless of the problem. Again, the data suggest that the nurses tried to take this approach. The nurses spoke of 'treating all the patients the same': 'You wouldn't treat patients any different, but what you would offer them would be different' (Jock).

Close examination of the occasions when the nurses asserted that they 'treated the patients the same', however, not only belied this but also showed that some of the nurses differentiated between 'treating' patients and 'offering treatment'. This demonstrates two different usages of the verb 'treat' ('I treat all my patients fairly' and 'I am treating so-and-so for depression'). Putting this more analytically, the differentiation showed that the nurses were talking in the first instance about taking a general caring approach and manner to all patients. This relates to the earlier discussion of the importance of 'showing that you care'. In reality, the nurses did not really treat everyone the same, and different patients were offered different treatments.

Downie and Telfer (1980) propose:

> 'What is required is that all differences of treatment be based on a criterion which will group like cases together and distinguish unlike cases, for *morally appropriate* reasons. In this context the obvious criterion is *need*, since the aim of proferring help is to meet needs: those whose need is greatest should get more help than those whose need is less, and those whose need is equal should get equal help ... We can call this requirement that any differences of treatment be based on morally appropriate reasons, a principle of *equity*. Equity is not the same as equality, since it says not only that like cases must be treated equally but also that unlike cases must be treated unequally.'

As we have seen, the nurses did not treat like cases equally, and different nurses came to different decisions in relation to what appeared to be similar situations. These examples showed that there was disagreement amongst community psychiatric nurses about whether they should undertake 'social visits' to lonely individuals. Some nurses argued that it was legitimate for a community psychiatric nurse to visit patients to provide companionship, friendship and social stimulation on the grounds that the visits prevented patients becoming depressed and mentally ill. The nurses, therefore, asserted that they had the moral foundation to continue visits. Other nurses argued that 'social visits' were not the legitimate work of the community psychiatric nurse when there were other patients in current need of 'therapy' from a skilled psychiatric nurse.

Again, we see how resource availability influenced the views and actions of the nurses. Who received what resources then became a moral question, and the nurses justified their input by reference to their training and to arguments which legitimated contact with non-mentally ill individuals (see below). The nurses had different ideas about what work should be done for payment, and some of the nurses argued that to 'drink tea' was not 'therapy', and that helping loneliness should be taken on by someone else, presumably on an unpaid basis. These differences of opinion about who should receive what care are brought into sharp profile because the resources available to the nurses are scarce.

The recipients of community psychiatric nursing care The community psychiatric nurses sought to justify their work by reference to their training. Some of the nurses argued that they were trained to deal with the mentally ill, not with lonely individuals. The data show that the community psychiatric nurses had a clear idea of what they were trained to deal with. An excerpt illustrates this point:

> 'I'd prefer not to take on injections. I don't mind psychotics, but not injections. I don't find job satisfaction with them. It is still a fair amount of my work, a big part of my job. I find it boring. I prefer the "vague referrals". I feel I am working as a professional, using my own skills to find out their problem areas. I am virtually deciding myself how to handle it, and I come to the decision of when to discharge. From that point of view, I am using my training properly. With the injections, it is just a procedure.' (Kevin)

Few of the nurses in the study had specialised training for community psychiatric nursing work. This reflects the picture nationally of a minority of practising community psychiatric nurses who have undergone specific training (see chapter 2). The interview data suggest that the nurses with specific training seemed to be less in favour of 'social visits'; it is unclear whether their training accounted for this or whether it provided them with skills which were better used with other clients. Regardless of possession of community psychiatric nursing qualification, all the nurses had a clear idea of what they were doing and why.

The following paragraphs present a brief theoretical discussion on the possible recipients of community psychiatric nursing care. Most community psychiatric nurses, by virtue of their hospital-based education, are trained to deal predominantly with diagnosed psychiatric illness which is severe enough to warrant hospital care. Skidmore and Friend (1984 a-f) offer support for this view and state that, at present, psychiatric nurses are not trained to deal with the less serious forms of mental illness. If legitimacy of work is defined by training, psychiatric nurses should, strictly speaking, be working only with hospitalised and recuperating patients with a diagnosis of serious mental illness.

This conclusion can be questioned. Many authors argue, for

instance, that the psychiatric nurse may have a valid part to play in work, not only with designated patients, but also with carers and families of patients (Falloon et al, 1984; Orford, 1987). Others argue that it is legitimate for psychiatric nursing work to be with non-nurse professionals, to transmit skills to other helping agencies (Goldberg and Huxley, 1980).

There is also a body of literature which argues that psychiatric work (in order to benefit the mental health of the whole of society) should embrace primary, secondary and tertiary levels of prevention (see chapter 2). This latter focus of psychiatric work includes work aimed at health education: primary prevention to prevent psychiatric illness occurring at all; secondary prevention by early diagnosis and treatment of illness to prevent and reduce the duration of disability; and tertiary prevention, the maintenance of function despite incapacity or disability. Secondary and tertiary preventative work focuses on designated patients, whereas primary prevention involves work with healthy individuals. Community psychiatric nurses can justify intervention with a variety of individuals by referring to any one of these preventative approaches.

These levels of intervention are not as clear cut as one would imagine, however, because of the confusion which can arise from debate on how the limits of 'mental illness' should be defined. Some examples demonstrate this confusion: should individuals in the community being given relaxation therapy by community psychiatric nurses for feelings of panic be labelled 'mentally ill'?; what about, in comparison, someone being treated with valium for the same problem? This confusion is compounded by the emphasis in contemporary psychiatric care on avoiding hospitalisation and treating people at home if possible. Is someone seen only once by community nurses 'during crisis' considered to be a psychiatric patient – he may not be diagnosed as 'mentally ill', yet he may have case notes in the psychiatric hospital? What about an individual who has suffered a psychotic episode, been successfully treated and is now well on long-term injections and attending day care – is this person mentally ill?

The question of whom community psychiatric nurses are trained to help is not easy to answer and is the subject of debate and controversy in the literature. The differing views, evident in the interview data, reflect differences of opinion about more general areas of community psychiatric nursing work, and about whether the job of community psychiatric nursing is that of 'primary prevention' or 'secondary prevention'. Bearing in mind previous comments about the work being aimed at the 'overall good' (of society), it could also be argued that the work of the community psychiatric nurses should be aimed at 'preventing' mental illness. Some of the nurses subscribed to this view and, paradoxically in the face of lack of resources, actually undertook 'work-finding' activities. An excerpt from the data demonstrates this:

'I'm trying to break down the image of the mental institution that the public have. I'll say, "Look, I could not help anyone in chains". I'll explain, as the image is terrible and mental illness is regarded with suspicion. My job is talking to and teaching the public. I was in a wee shop this morning and the girl asked what job I did. I said I was a community psychiatric nurse. It turned out that her daughter was psychiatrically ill and I said if she felt she needed me, to get in touch.' (Jock)

In view of the limited resources available to community psychiatric nurses, it is perhaps surprising that the nurses engaged in activities which added to their workload.

Despite debates about whether it is legitimate for nurses' work to be exclusively with individuals who have, or who have had, serious mental illness, the fact remains that many community psychiatric nurses, including those in the present study, are involved in care of people suffering from minor emotional stress. In view of the above discussion on training, questions must be raised about how nurses learn to care for these patients, if not in the formal nurse training school and colleges. This study shows that the nurses have learned their own ways of dealing with patients.

There is evidence from the interview data that mixed case-loads, i.e. of patients requiring primary and secondary preventative work, served the practical purpose of motivating the nurses.

'I'd get bored with geriatrics all the time. I actually quite enjoy working with anxiety, that is one of the things I really do like to do, but if I have done two or three days of just anxious patients, I like to do some with psychotic patients who are not a lot of hard work.' (Ivan)

This may be an important consideration as regards organisation of community psychiatric nursing services. Recent nursing literature on the concept of 'burn-out' demonstrates that professionals working in stressful and emotionally-demanding situations for prolonged periods can become 'spent', resulting in reduced work performance (Cherniss, 1980). One way of avoiding this is to provide varied, interesting and supportive work situations (Hume and Pullen, 1986). The above quote shows how variety within an individual nurse's case-load can sustain interest and enthusiasm for the job.

Psychiatric nurse managers in the community, at service level, must address the issues of what the community psychiatric nurse should be doing and with whom, and they should be making joint decisions about service organisation and planning. The data here suggest that these issues are not being tackled at local level and that individual nurses are left to make their own decision about who receives care. The DHSS (Department of Health and Social Security, 1975) recommended that local needs be used as a basis for local planning, instead of national criteria and standards being set for community psychiatric nursing services. This study suggests that local (mental health) needs are mopped up in a rather hit-and-miss fashion by individual practitioners, rather than being met by any planned strategy of intervention. Planning at local level seems vital, especially because staffing levels constrain or even determine the types of care offered.

The community psychiatric nurses in this study have clearly adopted many coping mechanisms and devices which have enabled them to provide a community psychiatric nursing service despite limited resources and infinite demands. These, in themselves, could be described as a defence against anxiety, devices which the nurses used to ensure that the service worked. These devices were learned in the practical situation, not formally in the nursing colleges, and were the means by which the community psychiatric nurses organised and planned their work with the patients. Gouldner (1959) commented on the 'informal patterns [of] organizationally unprescribed culture structures – that is, patterns of belief and sentiment', which develop among groups of workers in organi-sations. The community psychiatric nurses' use of labels could be described as one such informal pattern of behaviour. The nurses seemed to be socialised into what is legitimate by contact with their colleagues and peers.

The major control imposed on the community psychiatric nurses was 'finite resources'. These, in fact, restrained the nurses from totally 'doing their own thing'. This, combined with the checking-out behaviour of the nurses, resulted in the nurses providing a service which was remarkably standardised and uniform. The interview data provided an illuminating study of how the nurses made an under-resourced system function and of how they strove to make the service appear fair and uniform despite plenty of evidence to the contrary.

THE PATIENTS' VIEW OF THE SERVICES

The present study was motivated by a concern to find out whether the community psychiatric nursing contact helped families to cope with the burden of caring for a mentally-ill relative at home. The study focused on whether or not the community psychiatric nursing services met the needs of the carers. I would argue that the patients' needs should be the major rationale for developing services, but the involvement of patients in the present study was not to examine whether their needs were being met, but, rather, to gain feedback about their experience of the 'process' of community psychiatric nursing. This was valuable for two reasons, first, as an adjunct to the data received from the nurses who described their work – here the focus of concern was to obtain information on the 'process' of com-munity psychiatric nursing – and, second, in order to demonstrate an interest in community psychiatric nursing to the patients before asking for their permission to approach a carer.

This section examines the patients' view of the community psychiatric nursing services. As described in chapter 3, patients used the PQRST which consisted of statements on, and questions about, the helpfulness of the community psychiatric nurses. This procedure produced information on agreement or disagreement with the statements, and obtained answers to questions on a scale of 0 ('absolutely no help') to 9 ('a very considerable help'). The data collection took place in two different areas. There were two different questionnaires for patients, depending on the setting of the community nurse contact: day care or home visit (see chapter 3 for the reasoning behind this decision).

The text which follows presents a simplified version of the findings which resulted from the original study. The reason for this decision is that the 'discussion' was considered to be of most interest and relevance to readers interested in the topic of community psychiatric nursing and to novice researchers. The complete results produced by the study are available for scrutiny in the unpublished thesis (Pollock, 1987). There can be found the details of the number of patients who completed the PQRST, and a detailed breakdown of the items in the 'day-care PQRST' and the 'home-visiting PQRST'; the findings for each area of data collection are displayed side by side to enable direct comparisions and to allow for evaluation of the evidence of material differences between the two data sets. The avid reader and experienced researcher wishing to know this depth of detail are directed to Pollock (1987), available from the Royal College of Nursing Library in London or from Edinburgh University via interlibrary loan.

The results and the analysis
The patients were initially asked to agree or disagree with the statements in the PQRST (see table 3 in Pollock, 1987), examination of which gave an insight into how the care given by the community psychiatric nurses was perceived (see below). The answers to the statements were then analysed using descriptive statistics. In addition to looking at the answers to individual questions, scores of 0–4 were considered as 'unhelpful' and scores of 5–9 as 'helpful'; scores were also subdivided into three and more complex relationships were explored within the data. The chi-square technique was then used to test for statistical significance of the frequency counts of scores within the above groups. In relation to these, male and female patients, attributes of individual nurses and frequency of contact were tested to find out whether there were specific factors of the nurses or patients which affected helpfulness. Scattergrams were also completed for each item of the day-care PQRST to see whether frequency of contact was in any way related to helpfulness. In this

study, all associations below the 0.05 level of probability of occurring by chance (5%) were considered to be significant (different probability levels are, therefore, not cited in the text).

As described in chapter 3, the outcome criterion used in the PQRST, 'helpful/not helpful', derived from a range of scores representing 'no help' via 'a little help' to 'very considerable help'. A score of zero meant 'no help' and scores of 1–4, therefore, comprise the 'least helpful' end of this range. This distinction between helpful and unhelpful requires qualification, because it is not strictly accurate to characterise the less helpful end of this scale as 'unhelpful' for two reasons. First 'un-'adjectives like this tend to have a negative meaning, which implies that the nurses were actively un-helpful (the data did not suggest this). Second, it could be argued that a little help is a lot better than no help at all (a point referred to by the carers). This reservation about the interpretation of the findings should be borne in mind as one reads the discussion of the analysis.

A discussion of the findings from the day-care PQRST and the home-visiting PQRST is presented below. Patients of community psychiatric nurses based in East Hospital are referred to as 'East' patients; those of the nurses attached to West Hospital are referred to as 'West' patients.

The day-care PQRST

Only 'East' patients completed this questionnaire; all 'West' patients were visited at home because no day centres existed outside the parent hospital. Craig (1978) completed a study on day care and commented:

> 'This data shed no light on the actual quality of care provided for any one patient, its appropriateness, the importance or otherwise of maintenance of family and community supports for a patient or the removal or non removal of burden on family or community agencies.'

In contrast, the responses from the patients in the present study using the day-care PQRST do shed some light on the patients' perception of care, and on the quality of care given by the East Hospital community psychiatric nurses who ran the day centres. These responses are now discussed.

The results of the day-care PQRST

Looking at the day-care PQRST as a whole, the statements collected from patients in the pilot study (see p.87) could be broadly described as either 'nurse-', 'patient-' or 'situation-focused' (see table 3, Pollock, 1987). Most of the statements were 'nurse-focused'. Some of the statements classified as 'patient-focused' could be judged as 'nurse-focused', e.g. 'I made friends at the day centre' or 'I have company at the day centre'; on first reading, these appear to be related to the patients at the day centre, but it could be the case that the statements also related to the nurses. The items show that the patients talked about the community psychiatric nurses in the plural, not about specific nurses. It must be acknowledged that the answers refer to judgments about contacts with several community psychiatric nurses and may be undervaluing the helpfulness of individual community psychiatric nurses, although the converse is also true.

The fact that so many of the statements referred to the nurse, and that such a high percentage of patients found that the *nurse's* taking an interest, giving support, talking to patients, caring and asking about how the patients felt, was helpful, suggests that the *nurse's* being at the day centre was important. In the absence of a comparison group, however, it is impossible to know whether the nurses added something different compared to a day centre run by another profession or group. The nurses did not just 'talk' to the patients; there is evidence from the patient responses that the nurses' conversations were seen as helping patients to look at their situations differently, and that most of these found this helpful. Forty-one per cent agreed that the nurses 'delved into the past', and many found this helpful.

The responses from the patients suggest that the day-care service was seen as a place where they could discuss psychiatric matters, as the statement, 'The nurses ken about me' suggests. This could also be inferred from the statement, 'The nurses have special qualifications'. The answers to the statement, 'People at the day centre are worse off than me' suggest that this aspect of the day centre was seen to be unhelpful by 41% of the patients. Twenty per cent of the patients, however, were not helped by 'meeting others with similar troubles'; perhaps the fact that more patients were helped by meeting others with similar problems suggests that this could be a guide for future service development.

Different patients received different care at the day centre, e.g. group work, playing games or keeping busy, and these factors of the day centre were perceived differently. It is regretted that further details about these patients (e.g. type and length of illness, etc.) were not collected to find out what patient attributes are linked with this different perception of the community psychiatric nurses' helpfulness.

It will be remembered that the scores given by the patients were divided artificially for the purpose of analysis into 'helpful' and 'unhelpful'; this distinction should be interpreted with care. More weight should be attached to the patients' comments about helpfulness. For the patients' comments on 'un-helpfulness' or 'lack of help', one is left wondering whether the nurses were rated as such because the patient had no particular problem in the area of enquiry. For instance, 34% of patients did not rate 'making their own way to the day centre as helpful', perhaps because they had no difficulty in the area of 'getting about'.

The day centre was seen by half of the patients to have 'a nice atmosphere', to be a place 'to go' and 'to be kept busy', and by half as not being these things. Most of the patients found these aspects of the day centre helpful, although some did not. A high percentage of patients found the nurses' talking and caring to be helpful. It could be argued that it was this aspect of the day centre that kept patients attending.

Of the more complex relationships examined, the only associations that emerged as significant were in relation to the statements, 'The nurses take an interest in me' and, 'I made friends through the day centre'. The least experienced nurses in community work who took an interest were more likely to be perceived as helpful and were more likely to help patients to make friends. It is difficult to know whether this finding really does mean that the nurses with less experience in community work are more helpful. It could well be that other attributes of the less experienced nurses made them more helpful. This finding has face validity, however, in that one of the risks of emotionally demanding work is that there is a danger of developing the 'burn-out syndrome'. Some of the symptoms of this include 'reduction of time spent with patients, reduced availability for discussion and the professional [becoming] less caring, more controlling and less feeling' (Hume and Pullen, 1986).

The home-visiting PQRST

The items in the home-visiting PQRST (see appendix 4, Pollock, 1987), obtained from the pilot study, are predominantly nurse-focused. Looking at the content of the individual items in the home-visiting questionnaire, there are far more nurse-focused statements than ones relating to the visiting situation. The nurse-focused statements relate to the patients' perception of the nurse's manner, what the nurse does and the effect that the nurse has on the patients. The patients saw the nurse's visiting as a patient-orientated service, as indicated by the absence of statements referring to family involvement.

During the preliminary period of observation (see figure 2, chapter 3), it was noted that the community psychiatric nurses from West Hospital did not work from a day centre base. In view of the limited number of 'East' patients visited at home, it was thought that it would be useful to gain more data on home visiting and the community psychiatric nurses.

The results of the home-visiting PQRST
The answers to the statements were analysed using descriptive statistics, in the same manner as described above. The text below gives an insight into how the care given at home by the community psychiatric nurses was perceived.

Looking at the frequency counts of the scores 0–9, the distribution of the scores was negatively skewed, i.e. all the items were viewed as 'helpful' by most patients in both of the areas studied.

For both 'East' and 'West' patients, statements on the manner of the nurse, e.g. 'caring', 'taking an interest', 'asking how the patient is keeping' and 'making the patient feel not forgotten', all suggested that the patients saw these attributes of the nurses as helpful. This finding provides support for the work of Rogers (1957), who suggests that empathy, warmth and genuineness are crucial facilitating conditions in therapy.

The nurses' 'being cheerful' and 'cracking jokes' was perceived as being helpful by a large number of 'East' and 'West' patients. This suggests that the patients perceived the nurses as 'cheering up' the patients and that this was experienced as beneficial. It would be interesting to relate this finding to patient data and see if this behaviour was differently perceived by patients with varied diagnoses.

The nurses were perceived as doing different activities: 'talking', 'having cups of tea', 'looking around the house', 'taking blood' and 'giving medication'. It is unclear whether these different categories were to do with varied needs òf patients or because the nurses organised their work differently. Based on the preliminary observations and interviews with the nurses, the latter interpretation may be relevant. The nurses based at West Hospital did not take blood, whereas the nurses from East Hospital seemed more involved in medication-giving activities, a conclusion supported by the finding that a higher proportion of 'East' patients reported receiving medication.

Half of the 'East' and 'West' patients 'had cups of tea' with the nurses and found this helpful. This does raise the question of whether or not this was helpful because of the talk that went along with this, or whether it was the company and social interaction that was seen to be useful. If it was the latter, it could be argued that a person other than a nurse could carry out this activity. Patients reported the nurses as being special: they were seen to have 'qualifications in helping others' and to be 'caring'. Without comparative data, e.g. finding out what different professionals do during home visits, or finding out how patients perceive other professionals, it is unclear what 'nursing' *per se* brings to the care of patients.

Peplau (1960) argued that the nurse/patient relationship is different from a friendship relationship and said that, in the former, 'social chit chat is replaced by the responsible use of words which help to further the personal development of the patient' (Peplau, 1960). With these comments in mind, the finding that almost 40% of 'East' patients and almost half of 'West' patients agreed that they 'knew the nurse's personal circumstances' is noteworthy. Although it is not entirely clear what this means, the suggestion is that the nurses share personal information about themselves with the patients. Peplau (1960) has commented that:

> 'The nurse's biographical data is a burden to the patient who has no recourse but to translate the nursing situation into a social, chum-like one.'

Contrary to this comment, almost all the patients in the present study who did know the nurse's personal circumstances found this to be helpful. One cannot help but wonder why this was helpful, e.g. was the nurse seen as a substitute friend? The strong agreement found with the statement, 'the nurse visits the home on a friendly basis' suggests that this may be the case, and points to the importance of this aspect of the nurse/patient relationship. One also wonders why the nurses shared information with some patients and not with others. These features of the patient/community psychiatric nurse contact must be explored further.

A high number of 'East' and 'West' patients agreed that they 'got to know the nurse', yet a lower number of 'East' patients agreed that 'a relationship had developed' between the nurse and patient. This suggests that patients see these factors as two different activities; the findings from discussions with the nurses suggest that nurses see these as similar. A very high proportion of patients said that they could trust the nurses, but it is unclear what the nurses could be trusted with; this proportion did not tally with the proportion who agreed that the nurse can be talked to in confidence. It is perhaps a surprising finding that these proportions were not similar; it is also surprising that 36% of 'East' patients did not consider 'talking to the nurses' to be confidential. Future work must be aimed at exploring what patients understand by the words 'trust', 'confidentiality' and 'developing relationship'.

The scattergrams for each item for 'West' patients showed that there was a trend for increased helpfulness to be linked with increased visiting. This could be related to consumer feedback; i.e. the nurses more frequently visited patients from whom they received feedback that they were helpful. This would confirm the previous findings of Sladden (1979), where an association was found between a patient's deterioration and a decrease in visiting frequency by the nurses. It is unclear whether the patient's rating of helpfulness changes over time.

Patients' views of day care compared to home visiting

It is worth taking the opportunity to compare the contents of the day-care and home-visiting PQRSTs, and to make comments on the statements used in each. The obvious difference, of course, is that the day-care PQRST contains statements relating to other patients, confirming the fact that some patients find some of this contact helpful. In the day-care PQRST, too, there is more emphasis on statements which refer to helping the patient change, e.g. 'the nurses delve into the past' and 'the nurses let me see things differently'.

The home-visiting PQRST items emphasise the friendly relationship developed with the nurse, e.g. 'the nurse visits on a friendly basis' and 'I know the nurse's circumstances'. These differences represent differing views of 'East' patients where the items for the PQRST were collected. The 'caring' nature of the nurses was commented upon by both 'East' and 'West' patients and lends support to the importance of this in community psychiatric nursing work.

THE CARERS' VIEW OF THE SERVICE

One of the main interests of this study was to focus on the carers' perception of community psychiatric nursing, and their perception of help was the main outcome measure used in the study. The selection criteria for carer inclusion are detailed in chapter 3. Carers of patients visited by the community psychiatric nurses of both East and West Hospitals used the family PQRST which, it will be remembered, is divided into three parts (for further details refer back to chapter 3). These carers are referred to as 'East' and 'West' carers respectively.

As mentioned above, this section presents a simplified version of the original findings. For more detail, the reader is referred to Pollock (1987) where the number of respondents is detailed, a breakdown of kin relationships to patients is given, the results are presented and information is provided about the statistical manipulations undertaken for each section of the family PQRST. In appendix 6, Pollock, 1987, the interested reader will find the complete family PQRST available for scrutiny.

Analysis of the family PQRST proceeded in a similar manner to that outlined on pp.156, and the reservations mentioned there are pertinent to the discussion presented in the following pages. Below, then, a discussion of the results is offered; possible areas for future research are also identified.

Summary of the family PQRST findings

The major findings from the completion of the family PQRST by the carers are that:

- the carers positively evaluated attributes of the community psychiatric nurses;
- paradoxically, the community psychiatric nurses did not offer comprehensive help;
- the nurses were selectively helpful as regards patient problems and the carers' experience of burden;
- there appears to be some variation in helpfulness between individual community psychiatric nurses and betweeen the two community psychiatric nursing services studied.

Paykel and Griffith (1983) compared care by outpatient psychiatrists with care given by the community psychiatric nurse. Paykel found that there were no differences using the outcome measures; the main finding was that the patients receiving care from the community psychiatric nurses were 'more satisfied' with their care. This study suggests that satisfaction with the relationship is an important feature of the nurse/patient contact, and indicates not only that the carers are satisfied with the community psychiatric nurse, but also that they find the nurse 'helpful'. The community psychiatric nurse is not perceived to be helpful to all carers as regards providing help for specific problems or the experience of caring; nevertheless, the carers were unanimous in that they found contact with the community psychiatric nurse to be generally helpful.

The carers' view of community psychiatric nurses

Looking at the content of the 'nurse aspects' section of the questionnaire, the community psychiatric nurse is appreciated because of the service specifically given to the mentally-ill patient. Furthermore, the community psychiatric nurse is perceived to offer a support to carers which is ongoing and available at times of crisis. 'East' and 'West' carers reported they could 'call on the nurse', and that the community psychiatric nurse 'would visit if anything was wrong'; these aspects of community psychiatric nursing contact were considered to be particularly helpful.

Psychiatric nurse training emphasises the development of relationships with patients. The replies of many of the carers, reporting that they found the community psychiatric nurse easy to talk to and a person with whom they would talk about anything, reflect the view of the carers that a relationship of trust and care has also developed with the carers. One would think that this in turn would have led to and enabled sharing of problems.

Community psychiatric nurses and problem relief

Carers were asked initially to agree or disagree with items listed in the 'problems' section and, thereby, information was collected on how helpful the carers perceived the community psychiatric nurses to be with current problems. No systematic information was obtained about past 'problems'. Carers' comments suggested that problems had changed with time and that previous community psychiatric nursing intervention had been helpful. The majority of the carers gave the community psychiatric nurses low scores for helpfulness in relation to problems or the experience of caring.

Although most of the scores were low, it could be argued that to be helped at any level is better than to be given no help at all. This in fact seemed to be the predominant feeling of the carers who voiced concern that this research might result in withdrawal of the help they were getting. The nurses, similarly, were aware of their capacity to provide only limited help to carers (see p.135), and the aim of their work was to enable willing relatives to continue caring for relatives at home.

All patient/carer pairs were being treated by the community psychiatric nurses during the data collection. The rationale of the choice of sample should have ensured that a range of patient/carer pairs were chosen, each pair being at a different stage of therapy (see p.77). The low scores on 'helpfulness' may reflect the 'process' of therapy. In other words, carers may have rated the community psychiatric nurse as of little or no help because they were going through the 'pain' of therapy and change, and, therefore, perceived the community psychiatric nurse negatively. An area of future enquiry would be to compare respondents who have previously received community psychiatric nursing treatment with a control group who have not.

Bearing in mind the above-mentioned comments that many carers could talk to the nurses about anything, it was contrary to expectation to find that over half of the 'West' carers and almost half of the 'East' carers reported that they did not approach the nurses when worried. This may provide an explanation to account for the further finding that certain carers were helped, whereas others were not.

The reasons why only some carers, when worried, approached the nurses were not systematically explored in this study and can only be surmised. The personalities of the carers may have prevented them from approaching the nurses. Or, quite simply, the carers may not have wanted help at all (generally speaking, or more specifically from the nurse). Alternatively, the carers may have been receiving help from elsewhere.

Other reasons why the carers may not have approached the nurses may be to do with the nurses. The nurses, for instance, may have failed to make it clear to the carers what they could provide in the way of help. Comments of the carers, during the PQRST procedure, suggest that they did not mention certain problems to the community psychiatric nurse because they assumed that the community psychiatric nurse would not be able to help. If community psychiatric nurses intend to provide relief to carers (and this is a point which is explored in chapter 5), the onus must be on the nurses actively to seek information from carers about the experience of caring, and to further inform carers of the available help. At the moment, as the qualitative analysis has shown, the nurses tend to listen to the carers with a view to picking out information which they can use, and help is offered, linked to the available resources. The qualitative analysis also shows that the nurses' work is patient-focused and preoccupied with making the 'system' function rather than with providing comprehensive relief to carers' difficulties.

The study also raises numerous questions about the problems helped by community psychiatric nurses. What sorts of problem were helped by the nurses, and why these? Were these problems helped because the community psychiatric nurses considered themselves most able to help with them? In what way were the problems helped? Was the help received planned by the community psychiatric nurses or was it coincidental? How were these problems brought to the attention of the nurses (by the nurses themselves, carers, patients, or other professionals)? Did others' perception of the work of community psychiatric nursing, therefore, influence and determine the work of the nurses? This research has only made a small step in the direction of answering these questions and many of them still remain unanswered.

This study has given an indication of the sorts of problem which, in the carers' view, can be helped by contact with community psychiatric nurses. 'East' carers reported the community psychiatric nurses as being helpful, with marginally more 'patient' problems. 'Demanding carer's company' was a problem for which the nurses in both areas scored highly; with regard to limiting the demands of patients, or helping the carer to cope with these, community psychiatric nurses, therefore, could be regarded as especially helpful. For the problem of dealing with 'aggression directed at the carer', *all* West carers reported the nurses as helpful. This may suggest that West Hospital's community psychiatric nurses were skilled at helping carers to cope with patient aggression, although specifically how this was done is unclear. The data that are lacking, as regards problem relief, are details about 'how' the nurses actually helped, an area which must be a priority for future study.

Hypochondriasis and suicidal behaviour were problems experienced by many 'West' carers and few 'East' carers. Some 'West' carers considered the nurses to be helpful for these problems; it is unclear whether this positive feedback was to do with the more effective treatment offered by West Hospital's community psychiatric nurses or whether the nature of the problems was more intractable for 'East' carers. If the latter was the case, this finding may be support for basing community psychiatric nurses in GP practices (see pp.29 and 153).

The other types of problem which are helped (for some of the carers) are different for both regions studied; nevertheless, the problem 'types' generally fall into a category of 'typical' psychiatric problems, as would be described by the lay public. This may lend support to the notion that the carers are instrumental in deciding which problems the community psychiatric nurse tries to help.

For similar problems, some carers were helped whereas others were not. What factors were associated with 'helped' carers? Was this help related to the therapeutic relationship of the nurse/patient, to nurse variables (only length of experience in psychiatry and time employed in 'community psychiatric nursing' were obtained) or to patient variables (length of contact and duration of illness, for instance)? These data were not sought. Exploration of these links would be a useful area for future enquiry, and are essential in relation to making comments on the provision of effective services.

Findings in the family burden section of PQRST (which focused on the feeling of the carers about looking after a relative) also suggest that only certain aspects of the experience of caring were helped by the community psychiatric nurse. Examination of these items shows that the general difficulties and feelings associated with caring are helped for some carers. Certain aspects of the management of the patient are shared with the community psychiatric nurse (being 'on edge' and sharing worries about avoiding upsetting the patient), whereas others are neglected. One wonders why this is the case. As reported by 'East' carers, the more extreme feelings and experiences of the carers are not relieved by contact with the community psychiatric nurse. (This is in contrast to the 'problems' section discussed above, where extreme problems appear to have been helped.) Could it be that carers are encouraged to voice feelings that are socially acceptable rather than to acknowledge deep feelings of frustration, anger, fear, or misery? Or put another way, perhaps the carers are not encouraged to ventilate these emotions.

The findings, overall, suggest that 'East' carers do not find the daily drudgery of caring, or a large part of the 'experience' of caring, for a mentally-ill relative to be helped by the contact with the nurses. 'West' carers' findings suggest that the community psychiatric nurses may be more specific in the help offered, but the data from this area is minimal and little importance can be attached to the significance of the findings.

Patient orientation of the service
The 'family PQRST' results provide conflicting feedback about whether the community psychiatric nurses were viewed as providing a patient-orientated service. Almost one third of 'East' carers disagreed that the nurses came to see the patient; one presumes, then, that in these cases the carers perceived the service as catering

for their needs. No 'West' carers disagreed that the nurse came to see the patient, suggesting that this service was seen unanimously as a patient-orientated service; paradoxically, however, only 29% of 'West' carers left the nurse alone with the patient and only 23% actually felt that the patient needed to talk to the nurse. Perhaps, despite the 'patient orientation' of the service commented on by the 'West' carers, the service was viewed as a help and support for them; it may be that the nurses worked explicitly with both carers and patients.

Almost 30% of 'East' and 'West' carers did not agree that the community psychiatric nurses assessed patients. It is difficult to know how to interpret this finding: carers may not have understood the word 'assess'; alternatively, this may reflect the carers' lack of knowledge about this part of the community psychiatric nurse's work (Mayer and Timms, 1980).

Differences in the community psychiatric nursing services
The 'nurse aspects' findings suggest that 'East' and 'West' carers have different experiences of the nurses. More 'East' carers had unplanned visits from nurses and had day care arranged for the patients. The community psychiatric nurses based at West Hospital also arranged fewer hospital admissions; a higher percentage of carers in West Hospital felt that 'meeting on my territory' was best. What account for these differences?

The varied settings from which the nurses worked can partly account for these differences (see p.65). Additionally, the differences may be related to varied patients' needs; the lesser use of hospitalisation, for instance, by West Hospital's community psychiatric nurses may be a result of working with a patient population whose need for hospitalisation was less (the nurses worked with direct referrals from GPs and 'picked up patients at the first filter'; see Goldberg and Huxley, 1980). More 'West' carers reported that the community psychiatric nurse contact prevented admission and relapse, although it should be noted that high numbers of carers in both settings held the opposite view, therefore disagreeing that the nurses prevented either illness or hospitalisation.

It may also be the case that individual nurses held differing theories about, for instance, practice and visiting patterns, a feature brought out by the interview data. The approach of the 'West' nurses (as judged by the researcher) was one in which the affiliation to the parent psychiatric hospital was played down. The nurses also emphasised the importance of avoiding psychiatric labelling, diagnosis and use of psychotropic drugs, and stressed the importance of helping 'clients' to develop coping skills and to solve their own problems. This approach may have been perceived by the carers who appreciated the care given at home, rather than in the hospital or outpatient setting. It is fascinating that the two services seemed to have differing approaches and practices, and the factors responsible for these must be studied further.

Significant associations in the data
Female CPNs were found to be significantly less helpful to female rather than male carers, specifically with regards to helping carers to 'do the right things'. This supports the findings of the Equal Opportunities Commission (1984) which found that more help was offered to male carers by the statutory organisations. Perhaps the nurses, in common with societal stereotypes, considered that female carers needed less support in the caring role.

Carers who 'felt they had to take care not to upset the patient' were not helped by 'busy' nurses, i.e. community psychiatric nurses with large rather than small case-loads. Optimum case-load sizes are debated in the literature with few constructive conclusions emerging (Driver, 1976). The evidence from the findings in East Hospital suggests that the size of case-load has an adverse effect only on this one aspect of caring.

The finding that the association between patient problems and patient burden was very significant shows that relatives who felt that they were helped with patient problems were also helped to cope with the experience of caring. This suggests that community psychiatric nursing intervention aimed at problem relief should also be effective at reducing subjective burden. This clearly has implications for the training of community psychiatric nurses and for the use of resources.

Frequency of visiting
The basis for carer selection in the study was the frequency of visiting by the community psychiatric nurses (see p.80). The community psychiatric nurses who visited frequently were first compared with those who visited infrequently; the only item that emerged as statistically significant on the chi-square test was that carers who 'wanted to keep the patient out of hospital' considered nurses who visited infrequently to be less helpful. It may well be that this group of carers had high expectations of the community psychiatric nurses as regards visiting frequency.

The scattergram findings, linking frequency of visiting and 'East' and 'West' carers' perceptions of helpfulness, found that an increase in frequency of visiting was related to an increase in the perceived helpfulness of the community psychiatric nurses. It could be the case that the community psychiatric nurses are influenced by consumer reaction. The community psychiatric nurses, aware of being perceived as unhelpful, may have responded by reducing visiting frequency to these patients. Similarly, the community psychiatric nurses more often visited carers from whom they received feedback that they were being helpful. The 'West' carers found that the experience of caring was helped as much by infrequent visits.

Some carers feel helped by a few visits, others by frequent visits, from the community psychiatric nurses. What is clear from the results is that frequent visiting is not viewed negatively. For those carers who are visited frequently, it is unclear whether the community psychiatric nurse is rated maximally after the initial visit(s), the pattern of rating of helpfulness then migrating over with more frequent visiting. Alternatively, after the first visit(s), the community psychiatric nurses could be rated low, the rating increasing after each successive visit. To ascertain the pattern of change, rating would need to have been completed after each successive visit to the carer. This would be a useful area on which to focus a future study. The comments mentioned above, linking patient data with the feedback about help in relation to frequency of visits, are also relevant here.

The 'nurse aspects' scattergram for West Hospital had a clustering of ratings between the 9th and 13th visits (see p.248, Pollock, 1987). This could suggest that there may be a maximum number of visits beyond which helpfulness is unrelated. Further data are required to confirm this.

Further scattergrams were completed showing frequency of visits in relation to items in the 'patient problem', 'family burden' and 'nurse aspects' section of the PQRST, to see whether visiting frequency was related to helpfulness for particular problems, family burden or nurse aspects. The scattergram for 'East' carers for the item 'the nurse is an outsider' showed a visible tendency for increased help to be linked to increased visiting. This association was not significant, and some people were helped maximally with few visits. It is unclear whether this genuinely reflects the help given by the community psychiatric nurse, or whether this reflects the developing nurse/carer relationship.

Raphael (1972), in a study of hospital patients, found that patients were reluctant to rate negatively care which had been given. It is unclear whether carers are also reluctant to criticise the care received. This study suggests that they will criticise, but it is probably reasonable to presume that the dynamics involved in developing therapeutic relationships with patients are equally relevant to therapeutic nurse/carer relationships; the comments found in this study, therefore, may be understated.

THE GOALS OF COMMUNITY PSYCHIATRIC NURSING WORK

One of the reasons for examining the process of community psychiatric nursing was to explore the 'goals', as expressed by the nurses. The literature suggested that goals of community psychiatric nursing practice tend to be stated in imprecise and broad terms (see p.42), and that the available quantitative measures used by community psychiatric nursing services provide little information on which to assess whether or not these goals have been attained. The laddering procedure (see chapter 3) was used to explore the nurses' goals and to see whether individual nurses were indeed vague in their expression of them. It was hoped that the goals could then be examined using the notion of 'ultimate', 'intermediate' and 'immediate' goals, as described by Suchman (1967). This framework was discussed in chapter 1, where it was also indicated that 'values', separable from goals, are the principles which enable priorities among goals to be established. For this reason, the values and assumptions of the community nurses were also examined.

It was anticipated that the expressed goals provided by the nurses could be checked out against what the patients and carers said about community psychiatric nursing work in order to ascertain how far the goals of the nurses were achieved. The following paragraphs detail the goals of community psychiatric nursing work and compare these with the feedback received from carers and patients.

The immediate, intermediate and ultimate goals of the nurses

The constructs elicited by the triadic sorting procedure (see chapter 3 for an explanation of these terms) could be described as 'immediate' goals. This can be justified on the grounds of the theoretical discussion (see p.24), which focused on the importance of the nursing process in community psychiatric nursing work. After reviewing the literature, it was hypothesised that the community psychiatric nurses would use the nursing process, the first stage of which is 'assessment and information gathering'. The interview data (chapter 4) confirmed that these activities featured in the nurses' work.

Strictly speaking, the initial goal of this part of the nurses' work is to obtain baseline information. Elicitation of 'constructs' reveals headings for the nursing assessment and details the sorts of information which the nurses used to plan care. As such, the constructs can be taken to be immediate goals of community psychiatric nursing work. The laddering procedure was then used to explore the thinking underpinning the relevance of each immediate goal; from this exploration it was possible to examine the nurses' accounts of the work and to identify their intermediate and ultimate goals.

Each community psychiatric nurse was able, when led, to give a version of goals relevant to his work, and the findings suggest that there is a disparate list of values underlying the work of each community psychiatric nurse. The elaboration of the goals into a triadic hierarchy is not as clear as the above theory suggests; this probably reflects the difficulty of being explicit about the complicated life scenarios with which the community psychiatric nurses have to deal. Often there was not just one intermediate goal, but several (see table 3 for a 'laddered construct', using data from the present study).

The description of a goal as 'intermediate' was based on the researcher's interpretation of whether or not this appeared to be a 'step' aimed in the direction of achieving an 'ultimate' goal. Irrespective of how the goals were described, this analysis showed that the nurses, contrary to the expectations of the literature, were able to discuss clearly the goals in their practice. Table 5 below provides a summary of the values and intermediate and ultimate goals described by the community psychiatric nurses in this study.

Examination of the immediate goals

With the help of a content analysis (see p.95), the immediate goals were examined to ascertain the nurses' orientations and to see whether the constructs showed evidence of concern on the part of the nurses for the carers. The headings for the content analysis were chosen with this purpose in mind. The final headings used in the content analysis arose partly from comparison with previous construct categorisations reported in the literature (detailed below), and were chosen because the descriptions fitted the data. An attempt further to check the validity and reliability of the content analysis (by sending it to experts in the field) failed. The choice of headings, however, was sufficient to show the predominant focus of the nurses' work.

Bearing in mind the advice of Berelson (1952), definitions of the details of the headings used for the content analysis are detailed below (table 4). Appendix VI shows the constructs produced by each nurse, sorted into the headings used in the content analysis. I tried to sort the constructs consistently under a particular heading. The headings are not mutually exclusive and it is acknowledged that some constructs could have equally been sorted under another heading. For instance, constructs which mentioned 'family' in relation to self-sufficiency were put in the latter category, although they could have been inserted into the home situation grouping. For this reason the choice of headings is not entirely satisfactory.

The content analysis showed that the majority of constructs were 'patient-focused' and that the nurses seemed little concerned with the families' needs; additionally, many of the constructs showed that the nurses were concerned with medical problems. The findings may partly be due to the choice of patients as elements for the repertory grid technique (see chapter 3). However, the results of the qualitative analysis, which explored the usefulness of the constructs with the nurses, did not reveal a marked change in this focus of concern.

The content analysis also revealed that each nurse produced a

Table 3 Details of a laddered construct with superimposed interpretation of goals and values written alongside

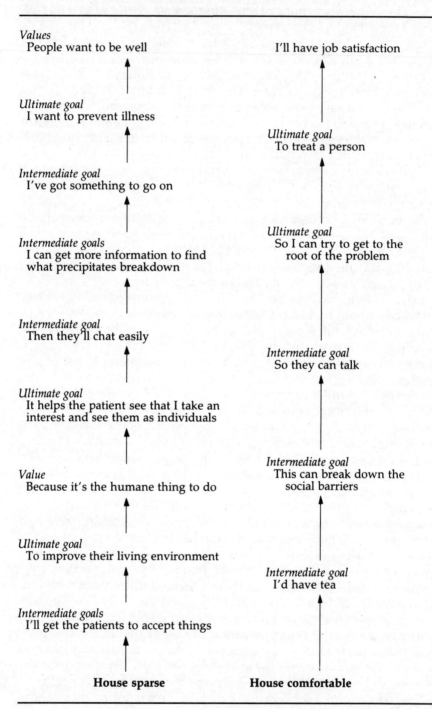

Values
  People want to be well   I'll have job satisfaction

Ultimate goal
  I want to prevent illness
                                                       Ultimate goal
                                                         To treat a person
Intermediate goal
  I've got something to go on

Intermediate goals   *Ultimate goal*
  I can get more information to find   So I can try to get to the
  what precipitates breakdown   root of the problem

Intermediate goal
  Then they'll chat easily
                                                       Intermediate goal
                                                         So they can talk

Ultimate goal
  It helps the patient see that I take an
  interest and see them as individuals
                                                       Intermediate goal
                                                         This can break down the
Value   social barriers
  Because it's the humane thing to do

Ultimate goal
  To improve their living environment
                                                       Intermediate goal
                                                         I'd have tea
Intermediate goals
  I'll get the patients to accept things

        House sparse   **House comfortable**

Table 4 Content analysis headings and definitions used

---

1. **Home situation**
   Any description where home situation is described

2. **Illness**
   Any description where illness label is used

3. **Treatment**
   a. Patient response
   Any description where patient response to treatment is mentioned
   b. Description
   Where treatment offered is detailed
   c. Medication
   Any description where medication is mentioned
   d. Time orientation
   Any description denoting future orientation or expectancy or past
   orientation or expectancy of patient contact with CPN services

4. **Social Interaction**
   a. Any statement in which face-to-face, ongoing interaction or lack of face-
      to-face, ongoing interaction is indicated
   b. Interpersonal statements which might curtail interaction with others or
      encourage it

5. **Work – finances**
   Any descriptions where work or finances are mentioned

6. **Self-sufficiency**
   a. Any statement denoting interdependence, initiative, confidence and
      ability to solve one's own problems, or the opposite
   b. The ability to attend to aspects of daily living – hygiene, washing,
      dressing, nutrition or inability to attend to aspects of daily living

7. **Factual description**
   A characteristic so described that most observers would agree that this is
   factual and not open to question

8. **Self-reference**
   Any statement where the nurse refers directly to himself

9. **Value judgment**
   Any description which is subjective and suggests moral evaluation

10. **Problems identified**
    Any statement where 'problems' are focused on

---

varied number of constructs, and placed different emphasis on the production of some types of constructs than on others (figure 12). The concern of this analysis was not to explore details of the working practices of individual nurses. The purpose of exploring individuals' descriptions was to draw conclusions about community psychiatric nursing work, both generally and specifically in relation to care of the carers. The findings of the content analysis indicate useful areas for further study to ascertain whether the differences in the constructs produced represent differences in the way the nurses used models or reflect varied theoretical orientations of the nurses; the differences may result from the varied contexts in which the nurses work, or may be related to differences in the patients.

The content analysis   Few category systems have been developed for construct analysis. Existing category systems were reviewed to see whether or not they could be used in the present study. Systems of categorisation have emerged from previous researchers' data: Davis (1984) used Duck's (1973) classification of constructs. The latter author classified constructs into 'psychological', 'role' and 'other' categories which, he claimed, allowed his constructs (on friendship) to be placed into exclusive and exhaustible categories. These categories seemed too broad to classify the constructs used by the community psychiatric nurses.

Philip and McCulloch (1968), using repertory grid, identified two clusters of constructs used by social workers to describe patients. These groups concern the degree to which a patient functions and copes socially, and the feelings of the social worker towards the patients. These groupings were relevant for classification of the constructs produced by the community psychiatric nurses, but were limited in that they did not enable description of the range of constructs produced by the nurses.

Lifshitz (1974), who studied the perceptions of trained and untrained social workers, developed seven categories from his work:

1.   task orientation;
2.   a description of concrete situations;
3.   abstract intrapsychic characteristics;
4.   abstract interpersonal or interpsychic characteristics;
5.   abstract social values;
6.   intellectual characteristics;
7.   affective–egocentric approach.

The categories developed by Landfield (1971) proved to be the most helpful in guiding the construct categorisation used in this study. Landfield developed a manual which provided 22 categories into which constructs could be placed. Some of these descriptions were borrowed: social interaction, self-sufficiency, factual description,

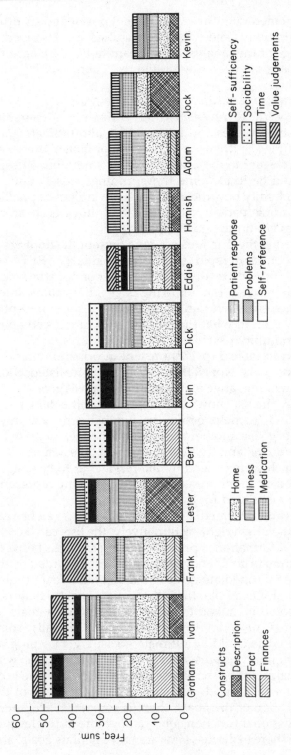

Figure 12 Constructs produced by each nurse, sorted by content analysis

self-reference. Combined with these headings, I developed six other categories. The definitions used with the headings are described in table 4. The findings of this analysis, the quantitative data-base for the extraction of goals, are presented in figure 12 above.

Examination of values, intermediate and ultimate goals
The laddering procedure revealed that different nurses also produced varied lists of values and intermediate and ultimate goals which, it can be assumed, influence practice. Elaboration of these lists for each nurse is irrelevant to the purpose of this study, but a useful future enquiry would be to examine these findings closely and, in particular, to try to identify how the values actually influence practice in the individual nurse/patient situations and how each nurse establishes priorities within the goals he sets.

The results detailed in the previous sections present the findings of the personal questionnaire rapid scaling technique (PQRST; see p.100) and, in effect, provide feedback on whether or not attainment of the goals was achieved. In the following pages, the values, intermediate and ultimate goals referred to by the nurses are presented and discussed in relation to what the patients and carers said about the 'process' of community psychiatric nursing.

The phrases listed in table 5 (p.178) present information on what the nurses said about goals. Not all the phrases used are listed; those chosen give a flavour of the range of descriptions of goals given by the nurses. For example, the list shows that 'to maintain the daily living skills of patients' and 'to help people be independent' are intermediate and ultimate goals; another nurse mentioned 'to increase the social skills of individuals' and 'to help the person take a more adult position in life', which were judged by the researcher to be similar. Different nurses used different phrases and the chart here represents a summary of the goals aimed for by the nurses.

The lists of values and intermediate and ultimate goals can be read vertically as lists in their own right. Alternatively, the lists can be read horizontally, as the information is presented using the links between intermediate and ultimate goals and values that were provided by the nurses. Some of the intermediate goals could be linked to a number of the ultimate goals; for example, the intermediate goal 'to maintain daily living skills' could be linked to either of the ultimate goals 'to increase independence' or 'to improve quality of life'. Equally, some of the intermediate goals could be ultimate goals; e.g. 'keeping an individual in the community' is presented as an intermediate goal, with 'to stop the individual adopting the illness role', but it could have been presented the other way around, and, indeed, was by some of the nurses. The classification of the goals, then, is somewhat arbitrary.

In assessing professional function, one can operate at the level of aims (the terms used here to discuss aims are 'intermediate goals' and 'ultimate goals') and take values for granted. This study has focused on what the nurses did (the qualitative analysis showed that the nurses used the resources they had to make the 'system' work), what they were aiming to achieve (the expressed goals) and an analysis of the outcome (the carers' and patients' view of the service, which gives an objective measure of goal attainment).

It is only when one starts to ask, 'Was it worth doing anyway?' that one gets into a political level of discourse where an examination of values is indispensable. At this level of debate, there are no possible purely objective criteria. In this sense, detailing values is less appropriate for the level of functional analysis, the concern of this study. The values of the nurses are detailed, however, as they provide information about the value base of the nurses' work, which influences the way in which the nurses prioritise the goal-setting aspect of their work.

The community psychiatric nurses could be described as working from a basis which embraces values to do with autonomy and self-sufficiency, preservation of a dignity and quality of life, respect for the individual and beliefs about care 'in the community' (for instance, that it is better to avoid hospitalisation and institutional neurosis and promote care in the family situation). As Downie and Telfer (1980) have commented, values are essentially comparative in nature, and this was borne out by the manner in which the nurses referred to values. The nurses commented for example, that 'autonomy is better', implying a negative comparison. The description of the values is related to the content of the ultimate goals. These values are displayed alongside the goals with which they were most often linked. As with the goals mentioned, this presentation is somewhat contrived and is not intended to be expounded as a rigid prototype but rather as a rough guide to the framework of values referred to by the community psychiatric nurses in this study.

Broadly speaking, the nurses' goals could be described as either patient-centred, job-centred or family-centred in nature. These though, were linked. If asked to clarify the goals to do with 'family', the nurses talked about helping the family to cope in order to improve the patient's quality of life. When asked to explore the importance of 'patient autonomy', the nurses referred to the importance of running an economic service or getting job satisfaction from seeing patients manage on their own.

Patient and carer feedback about goals

Feedback about the 'process' of community psychiatric nursing was obtained, and provided the substance of the statements in the PQRST (see chapter 3; and appendixes 6, 7 and 8 of Pollock, 1987). The comments made by the patients and carers have been explored

Table 5 A summary of the values, intermediate and ultimate goals described by the community psychiatric nurses

Patient-centred goals

Intermediate Goals	Ultimate Goals	Values
Improve patient coping capacities	Help patient to cope	*Autonomy*
Help individual to change	Help patient to manage	
Develop relationships	Increase confidence	
Help individual to achieve	Increase confidence	
Get person to talk	Able to offer self	
Give opportunity to improve	Promote independence	
Encourage patient to do things	Better to help self	
Discourage the sick role	Promote self sufficiency	
Focus on precipitants	Avoid hospitalisation	*Community care*
Help person to solve problems	Avoid relapse	*is good*
Set realistic targets	Avoid relapse	
Aim to work through feelings	Avoid escape to hospital	
Help person to deal with stress	Avoid escape to hospital	
Help person to cope with stress	Prevent illness	
Look for early warning signs	Prevent illness	
Get person to ventilate feelings	Prevent illness	
Provide company and stimulation	Prevent illness	
Avoid uprooting person/family	Reduce stress	
Keep people in families	Patient maintains role	
Keep person in community	Person won't learn sick role	
Want to get to know a person	Provide individual programmes	*Respect for*
Get information to work on	Provide individual care	*individual*
Show that I care	Be interested in person	
Be a friend to patient	Individual feels valued	
Get person to accept gifts	Improve environment	*Quality of life*
Reduce myths about mental illness	Educate the public	
Put support services in	Avoid risks	
Make self available	Prevent crises	
Help to give person a role	Increase self-esteem	
Help individual to mix socially	Feedback from others	
Help person to go out	See life is worth while	
Maintain daily living skills	Enable person to survive	
Help person to self-medicate	Opportunity to socialise	

Family-centred goals

Intermediate Goals	Ultimate Goals	Values
Develop respite services	Relieve family	*Family care*
Make carer's life easier	Reduce burden	*is good*
Give carer practical help	Improve coping capacity	
Help family to understand	Improve communication	
Improve home relationships	Patient stays at home	
Keep relatives informed	Family continue caring	
Give carer support	Family continue caring	
Allow carer to ventilate feelings	Family continue caring	
Prevent crisis	CPN and carer co-operate	

Nurse-centred goals

Intermediate goals	Ultimate goals	Values
I would lower my expectations	Avoid getting frustrated	*Job is satisfying*
Collect maximum possible information	Provide efficient services	
Get to know patient well	Use time well	
Avoid hospital admission	Prevent blocked beds	
Reduce myths about illness	Make job easier	
Educate public	Others' expectations fit	
I want to use my skills	Use my training	

above. It is also possible to look at the statements and to make comment about how the 'goals', as expressed by the nurses, were perceived and experienced by the consumers.

For the purpose of presentation, the statements included in the patient and carer PQRSTs are re-classified into the goals and value groupings used in table 5. 'Values' are included in this presentation for illustrative reasons only. The intention of this section of the analysis is not to fit the consumers' views into the same set of values as the nurses. This would be unreasonable: job satisfaction – a value of the nurses – could not be expected to figure highly in the patients' and carers' scale of values. The point at issue in this analysis is not the comparison of the nurses' and consumers' value systems, but, rather, the comparison is that of goals.

The major finding of this analysis is that some criteria for assessing the nurses' success in meeting their own aims have been fulfilled, and that there is a good deal of congruence between what the nurses sought to achieve and what the clients experienced.

The patients' view of goals

Analysis of the comments of patients at the day centres suggests that many are able to perceive the intermediate goals of the nurses (see table 6 which reclassifies the contents of the day-care PQRST in relation to the goals and value groupings discussed above). The ultimate goals were less accurately perceived by the patients; the most obvious omission is that the patients did not explicitly focus on the work of the nurses as being aimed at 'avoiding hospital admission', 'preventing illness' or 'keeping individuals with families'. Neither did the patients see the nurses as educating them about mental illness, although this could be implied by reference to seeing 'other people at the day centre being different'. A further point of note is that the patients also commented on the work of the nurses in terms of their activities; these descriptions could be likened to the task-centred definitions of community psychiatric nursing referred to earlier (see p.23).

Table 6 Statements in day-care PQRST, grouped in relation to the goals and values expressed by the community psychiatric nurses

Autonomy
I made friends at the day centre
The day centre is like a family
People there are worse off than me
I meet others with similar troubles
The nurses talk to me
The nurses have time for discussion

I talk to nurses about things I couldn't
    discuss elsewhere
The nurses let me see things differently
The day centre builds up my confidence
The nurses tell me not to get dependent
I make my own way to the day centre
The nurses delve into my past

Quality of life
The day centre is a place to go
The centre has a nice atmosphere
I can phone the nurses any time
The nurses give me support

I feel I am helping others
I am kept busy at the day centre
I get a meal at the day centre

Respect for the individual
The nurses take an interest in me
The nurses make me feel important
The nurses ken about me
The nurses care

The nurses say things that comfort me
The nurses don't treat me badly
The nurses listen to me
The nurses ask how you are feeling

Community care is good
I can get things off my chest
I have company at the day centre

Others at the day centre are different

Task-orientated definitions of work
I attend a group
We play games

The nurses give me my medication
The nurses arrange for me to see a
    psychiatrist

Unsorted statements
The nurses are cheery

The nurses have special qualifications

A similar interpretation can be used to comment on the perception of the patients who were visited at home (see table 7 for a reclassification of the contents of the home-visiting PQRST into the goals and value groupings detailed earlier). The patients visited at home discerned the intermediate goals described by the nurses, and the patients also focused on the task-centred nature of the work. Analysis further showed that the goals emphasising 'individualised care' were experienced most keenly. The goals grouped under 'autonomy' and 'community care is good' were comparatively little used. The 'home-visited' patients referred especially to the 'manner' or way in which the nurses worked; these comments could be converted into the intermediate goal expressed by the nurses of 'showing they care' or 'befriending'.

The carers' view of goals

Feedback from the carers about community nursing work was restricted to comment about the nurses rather than about problem relief or stress (see the discussion of the pilot study). For this reason,

Table 7 Statements in home-visiting PQRST, grouped in relation to the goals and values expressed by the nurses

Autonomy
A relationship has developed

Quality of life
You get to know the nurse
I know the nurse's circumstances
I can talk to the nurse confidentially

The nurse brings things I need
The nurse talks to me

Respect for the individual
Home visit gives better idea of me
The nurse takes an interest
I know I am not forgotten
The nurse cares

The nurse asks how I am keeping
I can trust the nurse
The nurse visits informally

Community care is good
Same nurse visits all the time
There is no waiting at the house

It is convenient at the house

Task-orientated definitions of work
The nurse has a cup of tea
The nurse has a look around
The nurse takes blood

The nurse gives medication
The nurse visits regularly

Unsorted statements
The nurse has other qualifications
The nurse cracks jokes
The nurse is patient

The nurse is attentive
The nurse is cheerful

table 8 presents a breakdown of the PQRST 'nurse aspects' section only.

One fifth of the statements in the 'nurse aspects' section of the PQRST refer to the patients (and are classified under 'patient-centred goals'); the carers, therefore, considered some of the nurses' patient-centred goals to have been realised. Especially, the carers commented on the 'talking' behaviour of the nurses. The carers were much less specific and less varied in their range of description of intermediate and ultimate goals than were the nurses. The nurses were considered to work with patients 'to prevent hospital admission' and 'to prevent relapse of illness' (goals not perceived by the patients). The format of the visiting situation was commented on, suggesting that the carers endorsed some of the nurses' comments about 'community care'. Again, what the nurse actually does, the activities of the nurses, were mentioned by the carers.

The remaining statements of the 'nurse aspects' section of the PQRST suggest that almost all of the intermediate goals expressed by nurses and included in the 'family-centred goals' list (see table 8) were endorsed by the carers. The exception to this was the goal of 'improving of relationships within the family'. Few of the ultimate goals were elaborated on by the carers.

Table 8 Statements in family PQRST grouped in relation to the goals and values expressed by the nurses

---

Family-centred goals

Carer can see nurse when patient is visited
Carer feels can approach nurse if worried
Carer feels can talk to the nurse about
  anything
Carer finds nurse easy to talk to
Carer can call nurse
Nurse will visit if something is wrong

Helps carer to understand illness
Gives carer backing
Tells carer he is doing OK
Makes carer feel less alone

Patient-centred goals

Respect for the individual
Patient needs to talk to nurse
Nurse comes to see patient
Nurse assesses patient
Carer leaves patient alone with nurse

Nurse can talk to patient and say things
  carer can't
Patient's presence inhibits the carer
Carer dislikes talk behind patient's back

Community care is good
The nurse staves off recurrence

The nurse prevents hospitalisation

Quality of life and autonomy
(none)

Task-orientated definitions of work
Nurse stops carer seeing a psychiatrist
Nurse arranges day care

Nurse arranges admission

Unsorted statements
Meeting on my territory is best
The nurses are freer

Nurse is an outsider
Nurse arrives unannounced

The 'outcome' information suggests that, objectively, the nurses did not help very much with a high proportion of the carers' problems. Nevertheless, some goals were attained, because some carers experienced relief of problems and help with the feelings associated with looking after a mentally-ill relative at home (see chapter 4). Many of the patient-centred goals identified by the carers were also attained – as evidenced by the high evaluations of scores given to the items in the 'nurse aspects' section of the questionnaire, as described above.

Before concluding this section, it is worth commenting that there is limited information about the nurses' goals which were not commented on by carers or patients. It could be concluded that lack of reference to a 'goal' means that the nurses were not working towards an expressed goal. This conclusion is not entirely accurate. Some aspects of the nurses' goal-seeking behaviour may, by virtue of the nurse/patient relationship, be misinterpreted by the recipients of care (see p.28). Furthermore, the goal, as defined by the nurses (for example, work aimed at 'promoting independence' – encouraging someone to go to the day centre), may be experienced as something totally different by patients and carers (for example, as the nurse showing care and interest). It would be unreasonable for all of the expressed goals of the nurses to be interpreted in the experiences of the carers or patients.

Suchman's statement (1967), that 'goals' (aimed for by practitioners in a service) should be reproducible, has been referred to earlier (see p.6). This analysis has shown that the community psychiatric nurses in the two services studied were able to do this: the community psychiatric nurses clearly detailed 'goals' which they aimed for. This is contrary to the information previously documented in the literature.

This analysis has also shown that there is a good deal of congruence between what the nurses sought to achieve and what the clients experienced.

SUMMARY OF THE STUDY

In this section, the work is reviewed, the reader is reminded of the original aims and objectives, and the findings of the study are summarised. This offers the opportunity to bring together material from the various parts of the study. Comment is then made about the limitations of the study and about how, in retrospect, the study could have been improved. In the final chapter, the opportunity is taken to look at the study in an integrated way and to examine its overall implications.

The work of community psychiatric nursing

The qualitative analysis focused on the 'process' of community psychiatric nursing, an area in need of systematic study. Drawing as it does on relevant literature, this analysis has highlighted issues relevant to community psychiatric nursing practice and revealed aspects of the way community psychiatric nurses work which were previously unknown.

It was hoped that examination of the 'process' of community psychiatric nursing would focus on the goals, assumptions and values underlying service provision and show how community psychiatric nurses do the work of community psychiatric nursing. It was also envisaged that the interview data would reveal to what extent 'caring for the carers' affected the work of community psychiatric nursing (see p.55), and would allow for the exploration of work with the carers, to see whether the nurses talked about 'reducing burden' or the negative effects of caring (see p.49), helped relatives and patients to deal with 'expressed emotion' (see p.52) or provided continuity of care (see p.53). The major findings of this analysis are summarised below.

The findings

Despite the difficulties of defining community psychiatric nursing and the context in which community psychiatric nurses work (see chapter 2), the qualitative analysis showed that there were common patterns to be found in the nature of the work of the community psychiatric nurses. It was difficult to sort the categories one from the next but, for the sake of explanation, three major themes emerged which pervade this account of community psychiatric nursing work. These were 'the ideology of individualised care', 'juggling resources' and 'justifying the care'. The nurses 'make' community psychiatry work by juggling with resources; they are placed in a situation where they have to compromise their expressed ideology of 'individualised care', and they manage to do this by resorting to various activities which 'justify the care' given.

The literature review shows that official reports on 'community care' are ambiguous and have confused aims. Some of this ambiguity and confusion is evident in the work of the community nurses, as seen by the confusion, at local level, over what should constitute legitimate work. Despite these ambiguities, the individual community psychiatric nurses were able to express clearly the 'goals' for which they aimed in their work (see above).

Community psychiatric nurses' work with carers

The nurses were more interested in the care of the designated patients than in that of the respective carer(s). This discovery was contrary to expectation, as the literature review suggested that the work of community psychiatric nursing would involve 'relief of burden' and offer specific interventions to families of schizophrenic patients (see pp. 51–53). The findings show that the nurses were in contact with carers, but the data suggest that the 'patient focus' of the work of the community psychiatric nurses should be emphasised. These results do not demonstrate that the nurses are providing care to the carers; any care offered to carers is secondary to and contingent upon care offered to patients. The focus on 'patients' at the expense of 'care of the carers' is influenced by two factors – lack of resources and how the nurses viewed the carers – both of which are linked (see below).

Lack of resources   In view of the lack of 'community resources' (detailed previously), the finding that the work of community psychiatric nursing was affected by 'resources' was not totally unexpected. What was surprising, however, was how strongly and crucially this influenced the nurses' work. Resource availability, or its lack, determined who the nurses worked with (patient or carer). Furthermore, the community psychiatric nurses appeared to offer 'individualised' care (as described by the patients). This may testify to the nurses' success in using their skills of 'developing relationships' by 'showing they cared' and 'playing the role of the nurse'.

Individual patients (and families) who did not 'fit' the available resources were variously classified (see p.139) and 'fitted' into a framework which allowed the nurses to legitimately, i.e. in a caring way, reject certain patients and justify particular care provision to others (see model use, below). The community psychiatric nurses, in effect, 'labelled' patients, an activity which prescribed management of patients. The data show that the sources of the demands (e.g. new, at risk, or manipulative patients) were the main determinant of who got what care.

The nurses' view of the carers   The data show that nurses view carers as a resource to help the nurses. This suggests that the nurses endorsed the view of care *by* the community, which was seen to be preferable to institutional care (p.18). The nurses' use of the 'independency rationale', implicit in the anti-institutional move-ment, can also be interpreted as evidence of the nurses' commitment to care *by* the community. Holding this view would imply that the nurses equate the primary carer with 'the community' where mutual respect and support was the norm (see chapter 2). This study shows that, for the relative, caring can be a stressful, lonely and isolating experience, as evidenced by the items in the family burden PQRST (see pp.238 and 240 of Pollock, 1987).

The nurses' view of the carers (which arose, in part at least, from lack of resources), and of patients (who were seen as individuals), also involved prejudice: the findings demonstrate that the nurses' preconceptions affected their work, although they tried to maintain good practices by developing a consensus and making joint decisions. Somewhat paradoxically, although the nurses strove to maintain good practices, other evidence, such as lack of the use of systematic assessment tools and lack of supervision, suggests that standards of clinical practice could be improved.

The interview data suggest that individual community psychiatric nurses had mixed feelings about the extent to which they should help the carers. The nurses were aware of the negative effects and 'burden' experienced by relatives; to a certain extent, the nurses' management of patients was geared to reduce this. Again paradoxi-cally, however, much of the work of community psychiatric nursing was aimed at maximising the help that could be gained from the carer. When the nurses talked of providing day care and social interaction opportunities, they saw this as being of advantage to patients by improving their capacity to relate to others (see p.26). This treatment was not offered as a means of reducing the level of expressed emotion to which patients were exposed, nor did the nurses talk of providing this care for the benefit of the family. The nurses did, however, talk of creating 'therapeutic dependency'. This shows the value which the nurses placed on providing ongoing support to patients. This term is similar to the notion of 'continuity of care' referred to in the literature (pp.53–55), although it should be noted that this phrase was predominantly used to describe work with patients rather than with carers.

One of the major findings about the work of community psychiatric nursing is the emphasis that the nurses placed on 'developing relationships' (see p.117). This behaviour was vital to the community nurses, allowing them to make the system work (managing crisis, preventing admissions to hospital and providing early treatment). This emphasis, and the nurses' accounts of the work, suggested that they used a 'social' model of care. The nurses, however, take an eclectic approach to model use (see chapter 2) and also used all the other models, namely the psychological, medical and behavioural. The nurses talked less often of using a behavioural model or approach. This emphasis of the work on 'developing relationships' contradicts the findings of other researchers who found that the work of hospital-based psychiatric nurses was based more on the medical model.

An evaluation of the 'outcome' of community psychiatric nursing

This study attempted to produce an 'outcome' measure of community psychiatric nursing: helpfulness of community psychiatric nursing input, as perceived by the 'carers' of mentally-ill patients looked after at home. The work of community psychiatric nursing was also explored, by examination of the comments of patients and carers about the process of community psychiatric nursing.

'Helping the carers' was emphasised in the literature as being a goal of community psychiatric nursing work (p.44). It was hoped that, by using the PQRST, this method would find out whether carers were helped by contact with community psychiatric nurses and whether or not the nurses specifically helped with relief of 'subjective' and 'objective' burden (p.49).This focus of the study was considered timely in view of the emphasis of current policies on the development of community care, which increasingly encourage families, particularly their female members, to care for mentally-ill relatives at home.

Systematic exploration of community psychiatric nursing work in relation to relief of burden has not been undertaken before. The present study has also examined a range of community psychiatric nurses' patients and explored 'frequency of visiting' in relation to outcomes.

The consumers' view of community psychiatric nursing

Chronologically, this study began with the patients' views of community psychiatric nursing. Both the patients and carers in the present study were able to give an account of community psychiatric nursing. The patients demonstrated that there were three strands which they found helpful about contact with the community psychiatric nurses at the day centre: these were to do with the setting of the contact, the other patients who attended and, finally, the nurses themselves. More statements were made about the nurses, suggesting that the patients considered the nurses to be particularly influential. Patients visited by the community psychiatric nurses in the home setting also made reference to the manner and attributes of the nurses, and to the benefits of the context in which they were visited (see above).

A major finding was that patients and carers found that the interest and concern shown by the community psychiatric nurses was 'very considerably' helpful. The nurses talked about 'showing they cared'; this aspect of the work was clearly picked up and appreciated by the consumers.

Another notable finding of the PQRST focus of the study was that the consumers' view of 'community psychiatric nursing' was 'shaped' by their experience of the service provided. The researcher found that the carers had little to say about 'problems' experienced. An explanation of this may be that the carers were unaware of the problems for which they could, or did, get help; alternatively, the carers may not have perceived their caring activities as 'problems' at all, but merely as aspects of the caring situation to be tackled on a daily basis. This interpretation would support the findings that the nurses 'shaped' needs. This conclusion can be linked back to the interview data, where we saw that the nurses controlled and manipulated the conversation with carers. These data also showed that the nurses were not predisposed to concern themselves with the carers' welfare and that help offered to carers was related to the available resources. The nurses could be described as 'ignoring' the burden of the relatives.

Comments from carers, during the PQRST procedure, suggested that the carers were instrumental in bringing up problems for discussion (see p.164). The onus, therefore, is on the carers to complain or raise problems – hence allowing the 'ignored' burden to become 'revealed'. Hoenig (1974) found that relatives do not ask for help; this is supported by the findings of this study, where half of the carers did not tell the nurses if they were worried.

The interview data also showed that the community psychiatric nurses used carers as a resource. The PQRST statements did not suggest that the carers felt 'used': in fact, many carers considered themselves to be supported by the nurses (see p.226, Pollock, 1987).

Feedback from the carers showed that they viewed the nurses as a crisis intervention service (in the carers' words, 'the nurses would visit if anything was wrong'). Additionally, the community psychiatric nurses are seen as a 'specialist' service where advice and expertise are offered on psychiatric matters. The nurses tended to offer selective help to the carers about 'typical' psychiatric problems and about the 'experience' of caring for the mentally ill, and it is unclear what factors are related to this selectivity.

Day care and contact with the carers

Cormack (1976) found that psychiatric nurses working in the hospital setting did not foster contact with relatives. Sladden (1979) found that the community psychiatric nurses in her study tended to have contact with the relatives in the home setting rather than in the clinical setting. It would be reasonable, therefore, to assume that community psychiatric nurses based in the day centres had limited contact with the carers.

In the present study, approximately 12% of the patients attending a day centre (7 out of 56) stated that the community psychiatric nurses had not been in contact with their relatives. This is further evidence of the nurses 'ignoring' family burden (by not visiting the carers of the mentally ill at all), a strategy which benefits the 'system'.

Limitations of the study

From the outset, this study set out to examine the effects of community psychiatric nursing work. The title of this thesis, although accurately reflecting the content of the following text, is not entirely consistent with the wish, also expressed by the author, to 'evaluate' and measure effectiveness. This inconsistency arose out of the difficulties inherent in evaluating a service as complicated and diverse as that of community psychiatric nursing. These difficulties, of course, are not peculiar to this study but are typical of any research work aimed at attempting to link outcomes with inputs.

The nature of community psychiatric nursing itself constitutes a whole spectrum of activities ranging from the one-off provision of information and physical help to a complex amalgam of practical and/or emotional support, counselling and collaboration with various agencies and professionals. The task of attempting to link change in patient behaviour with community psychiatric intervention might always be an almost impossible endeavour. In these circumstances, the 'natural' course of the condition being treated is unknown, and the question of whether any care is better than none will always remain unanswered. This study did not have any of the conditions sufficient to establish whether the outcome measures can, in fact, be linked to the community psychiatric nursing intervention, for example, random assignment of the population to an 'experimental' and a 'control or comparison' group, different interventions offered to each of these groups and clear specification of the types of intervention being used (with separation of the effect of the method used from the influence of the person giving the help). Bearing these factors in mind, the findings presented above must be viewed with caution.

Any attempt at evaluation is a matter of assessing the value or worth of an activity; if this is accepted, it follows the evaluations are, essentially, subjective judgments, varying with the viewpoints and the roles of the evaluators. The criteria used in this study to explore value were viewed from the vantage point of the families of patients visited by community psychiatric nurses. The carers' view is only one, though important, element in the constellation of factors that need to be taken into account in judging effectiveness. A fuller picture of 'effectiveness' may have emerged if other kinds of data had also been acquired which could have supported these measures. Furthermore, it should be noted that follow-up data are of little use unless comparison can be made with the state of affairs at the start of the intervention. For this, a prospective study would be required.

A highly structured measure – PQRST – was used to examine outcome. The aim was to produce as 'objective' a measure of satisfaction (of carers with community psychiatric nursing provision) as was possible. However, what could be said about 'satisfaction' remained very partial, and the data were difficult to interpret. The use of the PQRST to measure 'help' failed to shed light on what the carers actually meant by 'helpfulness' or to provide information about the reasons for the answers. Thus, the tool employed did not allow me to explore the thinking and reasoning behind the carers' views. A different research approach could provide these data.

Other reservations about the design of this part of the study include the fact that the number of carer respondents was small; this limits the generalisability of the findings. Nevertheless, the findings give clues as to the help that carers are receiving from community psychiatric nurses, and provide pointers to areas of future study. An initial intention of the study was to focus on a range of patients and their respective carers. It is regretted that more biographical details of both patients and carers were not collected in order to link helpfulness (or otherwise) with other variables. As a result, the available data are somewhat frustrating because they provide little information with which to explore the helpfulness of community psychiatric nursing work (see, for example, p.166, where the carers are selective about what they share with the nurses; it is unknown whether this is related to a failing on the part of the nurses or to a reluctance by the carer to talk).

All respondents were given a choice on whether to complete the PQRST. Those that agreed to comply with the procedure may represent a self-selected group which had strongly positive or negative comments to make about the community psychiatric nursing service. It is unknown how typical this group is of other available carers. Another source of bias in the data lies in the fact that all the patient/carer pairs were currently receiving community psychiatric nursing care; this may have inhibited the carers from criticising the nurses. Furthermore, the carers were aware that the researcher was a community psychiatric nurse. This too, may have had an inhibiting effect on the carers' willingness to be critical of the nurses. The findings, therefore, must be interpreted with care.

As with any piece of research, the endeavour raises more questions than it answers. The consumers' view of the community psychiatric nursing service was limited by the explicit focus of the study. Another research method, with a less structured format, would have allowed for exploration of the carers' views, expectations and past experiences of care provision. It might, in hindsight, have been more illuminating.

Any study committed to 'evaluation' of service provision should begin with clear statements of the aims being pursued by the clinicians. It emerged early in the study's conception that the aims of community psychiatric nursing provision were ill-defined; part of the study was, therefore, devoted to examination of the aims or 'goals' of community psychiatric nursing work. Thus, an evaluative purpose was in mind when the aims of community psychiatric nursing were first explored. This exercise became a main focus of the study, as it became apparent that the information had value in its own right and contributed valid data and knowledge about the work of community psychiatric nurses.

At this point, the researcher's interest deviated from being totally concerned with evaluation to a two-fold concern, with evaluation on the one hand, and with an exploration of the nurses' implicit goals and orientations to practice on the other. However, in keeping with the study's intention of 'evaluation', the goals expressed by the community psychiatric nurses in the study were subjected to close scrutiny. The statements of goals were, in fact, examined separately from the measure used to look at attainment. This raises two points which should be acknowledged in this section: first, was it logically acceptable to abstract the goals of community psychiatric nursing from the practitioners themselves, and, second, was it appropriate to compare these with independent statements made by patients and carers? Bearing in mind the earlier comments about evaluation of worth from varied vantage points, it must be said that this tactic only tells part of a more complicated and varied story.

Another issue which should be mentioned here is that of using the same data about nurses' goals both to define them and to assess how far these have been addressed (see above). Indeed, there is nothing intrinsically wrong with examining a body of data in two different ways, but there is also a circularity introduced into the argument. In reality, it is unknown whether the nurses, in the practice situation, did actually attempt to attain the expressed goals which they talked about in the interviews, and details about how these goals were achieved are also lacking.

The interviews were based on constructs gained from the repertory grid technique, and the interview format employed was that of the 'laddering' procedure (see chapter 3). These methods were employed because, as a novice researcher, I was not sure that I would be able to handle the data resulting from a more unstructured approach. This raises the question of whether the use of the structured interviews of the repertory grid, producing 'constructs', hindered or aided the collection of data on the process of community psychiatric nursing.

Initial response to this query would be to recommend the method, as tackling the interviews in this way forced the nurses to explore the information that they used. These data were previously lacking, and other researchers, using more traditional methods (e.g. Altschul 1972a, discussed on p.37), had found it difficult to encourage psychiatric nurses to discuss their work. In fact, many of the nurses commented on the fascinating nature of the interviews because they found themselves trying to verbalise aspects of the work to which they had not previously given thought.

Only a small number of community psychiatric nurses were involved in this study, and it is unclear whether the findings are generalisable to community psychiatric nursing as a whole. The findings do have a certain amount of face validity in that they appear reasonable to the researcher as a clinician; furthermore, the fact that the findings in the second site confirm the analysis in the first area also gives a certain amount of validity to the conclusions.

The merits of using the repertory grid technique were that this method made respondents think, and produced findings which have face validity. The method is heralded as one which enables exploration of the perceptions of 'individuals'. This was indeed the case; the strength of the method, as used in this study, was that the data were also successfully compared across the group as a whole. I would recommend that future researchers use this method in situations where respondents find it difficult to express their perceptions, and where the questioner's influence on the answers is required to be minimal. I have serious reservations about the use of the method combined with the rating and quantitative measures (see p.94), and would not support wide application of this aspect of repertory grid methodology.

There are, of course, more straightforward means of obtaining qualitative data, and it is possible (though not evident from any lack of co-operation on the part of the interviewees) that the structured nature of the techniques may have limited the ability and inclination of the respondents to enlarge upon their work. The use of the repertory grid method and laddering allowed only for scrutiny of the constructs elicited.

Pushing the nurses to explore the constructs forced them to think of generalisations which governed the work, although the nurses, in fact, often responded with comments on individual situations. Another method may have accrued different information, with less emphasis on general approaches and more focus on specific case management.

Taking a totally different approach with the nurses, for instance that of participant observation (see Pearsall, 1965; Spradley, 1980), would also have supplied qualitative information about community psychiatric nursing. With the benefit of hindsight, the use of participant observation might have produced useful data which are currently lacking. Thus, other factors which affect the work of community psychiatric nursing could be studied in depth; the influence of the multidisciplinary team on community psychiatric nursing work might, therefore, be examined further or, alternatively, an in-depth analysis of the nurses' expectations of informal carers might be possible.

In this study, the qualitative data obtained from the structured interviews proved to be the most informative and valid. In contrast, the highly quantitative data provided little information which clarified what it was that was helpful about community psychiatric nursing intervention, and data about the reasons behind the evaluations are conspicuously lacking. I would recommend that future studies on community psychiatric nursing work explore the merits of taking an observational approach, and suggest that use of such methods may gain more valid data than that obtained in this study using a highly structured and quantitative focus.

5 Conclusion

The findings of the qualitative analysis described community psychiatric nursing as analogous to the staging of a theatrical production (see p.115). This was because the emphasis of the nurses' work was on 'making the system work'. The community psychiatric nurses themselves 'make the system work'; this is with little guidance and direction, either from service organisers or from planners. Somewhat paradoxically, despite appearing to operate using varied *modi operandi*, the nurses provided a remarkably uniform service. These contradictory findings are not incompatible: they are testimony to the nature of the work, which is continually making compromises between the ideology, the resources and the care provided. The service appears to be uniform, because of the constraints of finite resources (which limit the number of ways in which the nurses can work) and because the nurses are socialised into the work of community psychiatric nursing by peers and colleagues.

The data show that the reality of community psychiatric nursing is that the nurses are not providing individualised care, but are, instead, continually having to juggle resources and to justify *post hoc* the care that they give. This reality has never been documented and, as such, must now be recognised by educationalists, managers and planners alike.

This study has shown that one emphasis of the nurses' work is on 'developing relationships'. This emphasis is testimony to the nurses' use of the social model in the work situation, and reflects the ideology of 'individualised care' used by the nurses. Use of this ideology is beneficial: it succeeds, to a certain extent, in making carers and patients feel cared for and supported, regardless of whether actual problems were helped. Service managers' future efforts should be directed towards helping the nurses to cope with the compromises that they are obliged to undertake in order to make the ideology 'fit' the resources.

The conflict that the nurses are in has implications for morale of the service staff. If the service is to be sustained and standards of care

193

maintained, these conflicts facing the nurses need to be acknowledged and focused on. This is not happening at present. Furthermore, what happens if and when the demands on the service increase – do the nurses merely continue, ad infinitum, to 'juggle resources' and 'justify the care'? The nurses should be obliged to take stock of what they are doing and evaluate where they are going. This study has shown that the individual nurses clearly express the goals for which they aim in their work; however, the community psychiatric nursing service itself seems to be unclear about its aims and goals. The future must bring better-defined services, which are clear about their aims and goals. To do the latter, the nurses will have to be encouraged to evaluate and monitor their work. This will require a fundamental change in their educational preparation, where there is an emphasis on integrating a research component with the work. Service managers need to address this issue.

It would also appear that, as community psychiatric nursing presently exists, the consumers of the health service are not getting the 'best deal' out of the service: help that carers and patients receive is dependent on the available resources which are rationed out by the nurses. The nurses used the carers as resources in order to 'make the system work'. Carers did not feel 'used', but the findings show that any help that the nurses gave to carers was secondary to that given to patients. Patients (and carers) who do not fit the service, as it is presently organised, are labelled and often discharged. Any changes in the work practices of the nurses or any developments (for example, liaising with GPs and working with early onset of mental illness) must be at the expense of care given to other patients (for example, at later stages of illness). Should these practices continue? If we are serious about 'caring for the carers', the work of community psychiatric nursing must be looked at to see who should be providing this care.

Focusing on resources also raises the question of who should be campaigning for the development of resources. The community psychiatric nursing service as it exists tends, consciously or otherwise, to obscure the reality of scarce resources (because the service succeeds in making the system work). This situation should be challenged and must be noted by politicians and planners.

IMPLICATIONS FOR THE FUTURE

The work of community psychiatric nursing

McKendrick (1980) posed the question, 'On what basis do community psychiatric nurses make decisions?' The study detailed here shows that community psychiatric nursing decisions are strongly influenced by the lack of resources and, at the moment, *individual* community psychiatric nurses make the decisions about to whom they do or do not offer treatment. Meetings tend to be used to 'rubber-stamp' these decisions, but do not appear to provide an opportunity for the nurses to debate and argue about priorities of service provision.

Lack of resources

The influence of lack of resources on community psychiatric nursing work has implications for the future organisation of community psychiatric nursing. These implications are relevant to the organisation of community psychiatric nursing work at two levels: first, at the level of community psychiatric nursing service provision generally and, second, at the clinical level of individual community psychiatric nursing practice. Each of these implications is explored below.

The organisation of community psychiatric nursing services

In the face of lack of community resources, urgent attention should be given to the issue of who should be receiving skilled community psychiatric nursing help. The literature detailing the theoretical arguments over who is eligible for treatment by community psychiatric nurses has already been presented (see p.152). In summary, these arguments rest on whether or not the work of community psychiatric nursing is considered to be that of primary, secondary or tertiary prevention (see also chapter 2). Also implied by the discussion were assumptions of what constituted 'paid' work, the inference being that tasks which could be undertaken by untrained workers should not be done by the community psychiatric nurses. These arguments reveal that community psychiatric nurses, theoretically at least, have a legitimate role to play with a wide range of people; the question at issue is whether the decision about who receives treatment should be an individual, a local or a nationally-dictated one.

Nurses within the same community psychiatric nursing service treated similar situations differently and, thus, held contradictory views about who was eligible for community psychiatric nursing treatment. It could be argued that different views within any one work setting are to be expected and are related to different expectations of the nurses about nursing work. For example, over 30 years ago, Habenstein and Christ (1955), described three 'types' of nurses: 'professionalisers', 'traditionalisers' and 'utilisers', who are in nursing for professional reasons, vocational reasons or simply to make a living, respectively. Nevertheless, in a situation of scarce resources, it would seem to be logical to ensure that the limited resources are being used in the most efficient manner possible. The interview data suggest that these differing views of community psychiatric nursing work caused some disharmony and disagreement within the community psychiatric nursing services, and it could be inferred that this was wasteful of the time and energy of the nurses. Having varied views of the work could, therefore, on one level, be argued as inefficient. Furthermore, the wisdom of 'using the existing resources to help as many people as possible' can be challenged; some would argue that it is more efficient to target resources to fewer problems, but to those which have clearly measurable outcomes. The managers of future community psychiatric nursing services should be tackling the business of who should receive community psychiatric nursing help, and should come to a compromise about who should be the focus of community psychiatric nursing work, instead of leaving the decisions, as at present, to individual practitioners.

The first question that arises from this comment is, then, 'Should *nurses in any one service* jointly decide who should be the focus of their attention?' The advantage of this approach would be that, as a group of like-minded peers, the nurses could argue for their respective involvement, using a common language and knowledge about nursing input. They could tailor their input to cater for local needs and problems (similar to the sentiment expressed by Department of Health and Social Security, 1975). If this expectation is to be realised, nurses would have to have an awareness of the contribution of other professionals and agencies involved in the care of the mentally ill. Demands in any one service are, necessarily, greatly influenced by the scope and nature of other available services, especially at the boundaries, as, for instance, in the care of elderly people, where the respective remits of the health and social services are blurred.

This has implications for the in-service training of the staff of community nursing services. They need to be provided with the opportunity to examine their work, to compare their working practices with other services and to update their skills in relation to clinical developments.

The community psychiatric nurses themselves may not be the best people to comment impartially on their contribution in relation to individual patients (see p.59). Bearing this in mind, it could be proposed that decisions by the community psychiatric nurses about who is treated may be more appropriately taken at a multidisciplinary level, where the combined views of different professions can be brought to bear on the work of community psychiatric nurses. The contribution of other professions may be preferable to the 'nurse only' decisions because others may be sufficiently distanced from the work of community psychiatric nurses to ascertain the contribution of community psychiatric nursing input. This study has shown that this does happen, to a certain extent.

This approach, however, may also have disadvantages. I have shown (Pollock, 1986), for instance, that varied organisational, gender, intraprofessional and training factors influence all members of the multidisciplinary team, and can raise barriers to the effective functioning of the team. The leader of the multidisciplinary team, often a doctor, may be the decision maker; this has been shown to affect community psychiatric nursing development and has resulted in referrals being controlled by a consultant psychiatrist. It results in the work of community psychiatric nursing being dominated by the medical model (Reed and Lomas, 1984).

This comment raises questions about the work of community psychiatric nurses (principally, whom should the nurses be helping and why, is the nurse the only person who could help this person, and, who has the expertise to provide the optimum level of care?), questions which, it should be noted, are equally pertinent to other professionals involved in care of the mentally ill. Additionally, any decision about community psychiatric nursing involvement will have implications for the work of others. As such, it could be argued that the issue of who should be cared for by community psychiatric nurses should be debated much more widely, by professionals, policy makers and voluntary organisations alike. This is a solution proposed by Drucker, who commented that the 'All Wales Strategy' provided evidence of 'the progress which can be made when the efforts of families, professionals, civil servants and politicians can be harnessed together' (Drucker, 1987).

Examination of 'work' usually means examination of the individual professionals and staff 'at work'. Policy documents – for example, Scottish Home and Health Department, 1985 (and this research study) – do not start with an examination of tasks, but of the staff involved. In future, we should be looking at what tasks need to be done for patients and carers – from the diagnosis of rare conditions to the support of those re-learning skills lost through illness, e.g. cooking, shopping and self-care, and from research into different treatment approaches to the daily physical care of those with dementia. Only then can we think through what skills and staff are needed to carry out the tasks. Future work needs to be done in this area, so that the most appropriate worker can carry out the necessary action for patients and carers. Information for carers of patients suffering from schizophrenia or dementia may, for example, be better given by peripatetic information-givers; company and social activity may be equally well provided, for patients who need this, by lay workers who are taught about and given an understanding of mental illness.

Each profession engaged in the mental health field has its own amalgam of knowledge based on medical and social sciences, and each has a tendency to claim individual coherence and authority. Yet, there appear to be difficulties of seeing, in practice, where the contribution of one professional ends and that of another begins. This takes us into the realm of 'role blurring', where there is overlap of skills amongst the professions.

The concept of the 'key worker' seems to have emerged because of this; here, an individual worker co-ordinates and organises the care of a patient (or group of patients). The profession of the worker is largely irrelevant, but what is important is that the key worker has the skills, abilities and motivation to help the patient. The key worker approach to patient care appears to make individual workers feel especially valued, partly because they have a clearly defined task which they are responsible for carrying out. There is also less emphasis on roles prescribed by training and power positions. Perhaps we should be looking at this area more carefully and, if possible, enabling people with less training to do certain tasks instead of overburdening the elite, like community psychiatric nurses, of whom there are too few.

Some work comparing the contributions of different professionals has already been done. Controlled studies have been conducted which suggest that social worker attachment to general practice has resulted in chronic neurotics showing improved psychological and social adjustment and receiving fewer prescriptions (Cooper et al, 1975). Marks (1985) found that psychiatric nurse therapists in primary care have been effective. These are psychiatric nurses trained to assess patients systematically and to carry out behaviour and cognitive therapy programmes and social skills groups – traditionally work carried out exclusively by clinical psychologists. Paykel and Griffith (1983) found that community psychiatric nurses were equally effective in the treatment of neurotic patients as were psychiatrists seeing them on an outpatient basis. These studies need to be replicated on a wider scale. It is only when this has been achieved that manpower targets, for community psychiatric nursing services, for example, can be established with any certainty.

The future, for community psychiatric nursing in particular, and for care of the mentally ill in general, must be one in which 'evaluation' of practice is a strong component. Drucker (1987) stated:

'Evaluation is a skilled task in its own right and not something which can be tacked on to the job of an already harassed project worker... More [money] should be spent on evaluating services and, if good proposals are not coming forward from outside researchers, the Scottish Office should consider commissioning research directly or employing their own researcher to carry it out. Furthermore, some of this activity should take the form of action research – in which projects would be set up with the conscious objective of providing a model for testing.'

This comment should be heeded both by the Scottish Office, which has a crucial role in encouraging the evaluation of projects focusing on care of the mentally ill, and by service managers who may be in a position to employ researchers to evaluate service provision. I have argued above for the need for evaluation of community psychiatric nursing services, particularly in the face of services functioning in a situation of 'lack of resources'. Even if the resources available for care of the mentally ill are increased, this argument still stands.

Organisation at clinical level of community psychiatric nursing work
The lack of resources, which, of course, includes community psychiatric nursing personnel, means that the work of the community psychiatric nurses should be examined to ensure that the 'best' use of the scarce resources is being achieved. This entails 'evaluation' of the work at service level. Additionally, the manner in which the nurses manage their case-loads and the influences of the individual nurses' practices should be explored to ensure high standards of nursing practice and efficient use of resources.

Clinical supervision   The aims of 'clinical supervision' have been detailed as being:

> 'to facilitate the nurse in developing a different perspective on her work with clients, by encouraging greater self-awareness and building strengths and therapeutic and coping skills. As a process, effective supervision is educative without being didactic, since it promotes learning, and increases confidence and problem-solving skills in a supportive setting.' (Simmons and Brooker, 1986)

This component of clinical work is advocated as a means by which individual nursing practices can be examined and can offer opportunity for the nurses to monitor, explore and, if necessary, change their practice.

There is plenty of evidence from the data that the practice of community psychiatric nursing would benefit from 'clinical supervision'. The organisational control exerted by the community psychiatric nurse managers in this study was minimal, although it imposed some safeguards on the current system of 'patient' and 'carer' triage operated by the nurses. The nurses, however, had plenty of scope to do what they wanted.

Previous research focusing on the skills of psychiatric nursing (McIlwaine, 1980; Cormack, 1983) suggested that psychiatric nurses in the hospital setting often take a 'medical model' role, support the work of doctors and use interpersonal skills minimally. The findings from the present study suggest that the nurses use various models (especially the social model with an emphasis on 'developing relationships') in community work. It could be argued that the community context allows the nurses to 'develop relationships' whereas, in the hospital setting, the time-limited situation and the urgency of the patient's condition restrict the opportunities of the nurse to focus on this aspect of the work. The fact that the community psychiatric nurses' work is so different from that of hospital-based nurses may indicate that this area of the work would benefit from the support offered by supervision.

The interview data highlight two other features of community psychiatric nursing practice which could be improved by the introduction of clinical supervision. First, the data suggest that community psychiatric nurses may have some difficulty in sustaining relationships: patients who are 'difficult', 'too demanding' or who become 'over-involved' tend to be rejected (see p.141). Some of the nurses, then, appear unable to handle these patients. Perhaps the opportunity for clinical supervision of psychiatric nurses' work would provide the support that the nurses need to be better able to cope with these 'difficult and demanding' patients. Secondly, the finding that the nurses have preconceptions of patients and carers is a factor of the work which could be explored and revealed during supervision sessions. This would be one, constructive way of tackling the issue of 'problematic' patients. In the light of the previous discussion, the matching of patient needs with professional expertise and, indeed, the whole issue of ascertaining the 'success' (or otherwise) of interventions, is an endeavour which is in its infancy. Merely introducing supervision is not the whole answer, but it is a step in the right direction.

Clinical supervision can be undertaken on a group basis, e.g. peer review or on a one-to-one basis (Community Psychiatric Nurses Association, 1985d). The former method of sharing of problems took place in an informal way in the services studied. If individual 'clinical supervision' is introduced into the day-to-day work of the community psychiatric nurses, one cannot help but ask who is in the best position to undertake this supervision. The easiest answer to give would be to propose the manager of the community psychiatric nursing service. Equally, however, it could be argued that another professional could do this work. Taking the notion of the 'key worker' concept (mentioned above), the professional with the appropriate skills should do the supervision (e.g. a clinical psychologist or behaviour therapy nurse if the nurse is using a behavioural model, a psychoanalyst if the nurse is using a psychological model, a social worker if the nurse is using a social model, and so on). If nurses are eclectic in their approach to their work, why should they not be eclectic in their choice of supervisors?

The attraction of 'clinical supervision' is summed up thus:

'It would be misleading to imply that systems of supervision and workload monitoring only benefit individual CPNs [community psychiatric nurses]. They can also be extremely important for the service in providing a forum for examining the degree of fit between the direction in which a CPN's work is going and the overall strategy for the development of the service as a whole.' (Simmons and Brooker, 1986)

This comment may indeed be persuasive in enticing the local manager to supervise community psychiatric nursing staff. It links individual work practices with the overall development of community psychiatric nursing services and takes us full circle to the importance of developing a strategy (see p.42) and of who should be targetted to receive community psychiatric nursing care.

Regardless of the debate about who should receive treatment from community psychiatric nurses, one would have thought that there should be standardisation in relation to certain aspects of care, at least in agreed direction of patients to service provision, particularly when resources are limited. The data suggest that there are some agreed ways of managing patients (e.g. not to follow up psychogeriatric patients, see p.150). Other approaches could be agreed upon. Fisch et al (1982) propose 'tactics of change' or options for 'doing therapy briefly' which could be a legitimate way of working in an environment of limited resources. In an under-resourced field, these options should be explored by both clinicians and their managers. This brings us to another topic relevant to the future of community psychiatric nursing services, that of training.

The work of community psychiatric nursing: training implications

Changes or improvements in clinical practice cannot be mentioned without comment on the importance of training aimed at updating and improving therapeutic activity. This has been implied by the above comments about supervision, and in the discussion about the knowledge base from which community psychiatric nurses would argue to care for specific individuals in the community.

The majority of community psychiatric nurses nationally (Community Psychiatric Nurses Association, 1985b), and most of those in the present study, are not specifically trained for community work. This study shows that few differences emerged between the trained and untrained nurses in the study. Nurses with the community psychiatric nursing qualification, however, had negative views about 'social visiting' (see p.123); this view may have resulted from the post-registration training which, it could be speculated, might have encouraged nurses to be critical of their work. The evidence from this study showed that, regardless of training received, the way in which the community psychiatric nurses structure their work, and make the system function, is by using a schema not directly imposed by training.

The data suggest that the way in which the community psychiatric nurses function is the product of a coping strategy, and demonstrate how the nurses make the system work. 'Clinical supervision' could be included in the future work of community psychiatric nurses in order to help them cope and function better. Alternative strategies could be taught to the nurses, such as using a behavioural approach to care or integrating 'systematic assessment tools' into the practice of community psychiatric nursing, each of which are detailed below.

The nurses in the present study said little about interventions which could be subsumed under the description of offering a 'behavioural' model or approach to care. Some of the nurses referred to 'goals' or 'target setting' (see p.123), and behaviour was focused on with a view to changing it (see p.127) but, more often than not, alternative models were used as the treatment of choice. The behavioural model offers opportunity for nurses to be systematic and focused in their approach (see above, and particularly the work of Barker and Fraser, 1985). This approach would be particularly advantageous to community psychiatric nurses if we consider the previous comments about evaluation and efficiency.

The interview data suggest that the nurses 'labelled' patients, and that this activity may have had the effect of making 'dependent' patients even more dependent (see pp.139–142). A more productive stance for the nurses to take would be for them to use positive descriptions, which may serve to motivate and promote patient independence, and which would also help the nurses to focus on the patients' merits, rather than on their deficits and demands. This approach has its roots in the behavioural model; nurses using this more positive focus have been described as taking a 'constructional' approach to patient care (Barker, 1986, Barrowclough and Fleming, 1986). The behavioural model, then, should be taught to community psychiatric nurses as a valuable approach to care.

An additional way in which teaching could potentiate the individual nurses' practices would be to inform the nurses of the benefits of 'systematic tools' (see Barker, 1986) which can aid focusing on the patient and can target nursing activities. These 'tools' not only provide a clear picture of the work to be done, but also form a record of interventions, which can be useful in the objective assessment of improvement or change. Systematic assessment tools should be used to limit the wasteful use of nursing input and to optimise resource use. Use of these tools would also be a practical help to the nurses when they have to make choices about whom to target for treatment.

Literature-based evidence suggests that some community psychiatric nurses work with patients with early symptoms of mental illness. Stanfield (1984) has described the use of the 'general health questionnaire' by community psychiatric nurses. This screening tool, devised by Goldberg (1978), provides a method of identifying emotionally-distressed individuals. If used by community psychiatric nurses attached to a health centre or GP practice, this tool can 'weed out the potential victims and provide prompt and effective service' (Stanfield, 1984).

The data do not suggest that the nurses were aware of the literature on expressed emotion (see p.52) and on the importance of reducing patient contact with carers (to reduce risk of relapse), although the nurses did speak of reducing 'burden'. These topics should be known by the nurses, regardless of the involvement that they have with the carers (see below), and they highlight another area of teaching which should be made known to community psychiatric nurses.

The previous paragraphs have identified specific research findings and practical techniques which should be taught to community psychiatric nurses. The issue of 'mandatory' training for community psychiatric nurses is a contentious issue, and the courses that do exist have been criticised because they do not provide skills-based programmes (see p.57). The above discussion suggests that community psychiatric nurses need more skills, and that current community psychiatric nursing courses should have a component on 'skill acquisition'. It could also be argued, based on this analysis of the work of community psychiatric nurses, that present post-registration training should be focused more on issues relating to coping with conflicting demands and to resource management, and should include a component on 'moral philosophy', for example, which may help to make these decisions better understood.

In relation to the 'mandatory training' debate, however, it could be argued that the required skills could and should be taught on an 'in-service' basis. This would support the philosophy of continuing education for nurses in Scotland, proposed by Auld (Scottish Home and Health Department, 1981), and would be even more applicable in the future if the proposals of the nurses' governing body, the United Kingdom Central Council (UKCC), for revisions of basic nursing education are accepted (United Kingdom Central Council, 1985).

The UKCC have published discussion documents on the future of the nursing profession, in which they advocate a more balanced mix of services with a shift away from hospital-centred health care to an emphasis on health promotion and prevention. The papers also argue that basic nurse training must be revised to accommodate the changes in orientation of practice. They recommend and emphasise a 'common core' training for all nurses, with a focus on the social sciences and the study of behaviour, life-styles, human development, concepts of health, self-care and coping mechanisms (where illness is considered to be a deviation from health). This is similar to the proposals of the Psychiatric Nurses Association in Scotland (1986), and is a departure from the current training which is bedded in the biological sciences. The proposed 'common core' resembles the content of present-day community psychiatric nursing courses so, with the passage of time, post-registration training for community psychiatric nurses, as we know it today, will become redundant.

Future community psychiatric nurse training may evolve to become skills-based training provided at 'in-service' level; if this is the case, training for community psychiatric nursing will not be specialised, but will be provided to all psychiatric nurses, who may in the future be doing more work in the community anyway, if the recommendations of the SHAPE Report (Scottish Home and Health Department, 1980b), come to fruition.

Community psychiatric nursing and care of the carers

One of the concerns of this study is community psychiatric nursing work and the carers; a final comment, therefore, must be made about the role of community psychiatric nurses with carers. Hunter (1978) commented that 'more active and open co-operation should be sought from the care-givers'. The present study suggests that the nurses do co-operate with the care-givers and, in particular, that the latter help the nurses in their work with patients. The interviews suggest that the focus of concern of the nurses is the patients and that this is partly due to limited resources. This is as good a reason as any to argue against increased community psychiatric involvement with carers. It could also be argued that community psychiatric nurses, as presently trained and organised, are not equipped to care for the needs of families and carers, and that the emphasis of their training is on patients' needs.

Teaching the nurses about the theory of burden and strategies to reduce the adverse effects (as proposed above) may go some way towards influencing community psychiatric nursing practice to encourage the nurses to enquire into the experiences of the carers as regards 'objective' and 'subjective' burden. The nurses may be then, if not able to treat carers, at least in a position to argue for service development based on 'caring for the carers'. This will put a stop to the current situation of the carers having to ask for help.

The importance, therapeutically, of the personality and attitude of the nurse has already been discussed (see chapter 2). The findings from the PQRST part of the study suggest that this component of the nurse/patient or nurse/carer relationship was found *maximally helpful*. The emphasis, given in the training of psychiatric nurses, on the importance of these attributes for nurses should be continued. The help provided by the nurses should not be underestimated, and many carers in the study commented that they would not know where to turn if they were no longer to get the help that they did from the community psychiatric nurses. The carers considered the nurses to be the key professionals in the community setting, whom they would seek out to get help with psychiatric matters. Unlike other professionals, for example, the community psychiatric nurses appeared to be available and willing to visit in times of emergency.

In the absence of improved, skills-based training for community psychiatric nurses, increased support to carers should logically be undertaken by another profession (for example, social workers). Social workers are specifically trained to do family work, and, as such, they may be able to take a more focused approach to their needs. The disadvantage of social work involvement in caring for the carers is that, until recently, under the guise of mental health officer training, they were not specifically trained in care of the mentally ill (Drucker, 1987). Having a social worker targetted to 'care for the carer' could result in two sets of workers going into a home, one to help the patient, the other, the carers. This may not necessarily be a bad idea, but it would be wasteful of resources, and would compound the split of 'social care' from 'health care' (see p.16), an approach which seems to be divisive rather than cohesive.

A more constructive and practical solution to the issue of caring for the carers would be for more research to be commissioned, aimed at comparing the contribution of different workers with varied expertise and training. Additionally, extensive surveys need to be undertaken focusing on the tasks that carers require to be done to help them in the business of caring for a mentally-ill person at home. Only then will we be in a position to plan how future services can be organised to the benefit of the 'informal carers'. This will be preferable to the current situation, as evidenced by the PQRST data which suggest that the community psychiatric nurses 'shape' the needs of the carers and (often inadvertently) render their burden 'ignored' rather than 'revealed'.

In focusing on the future of community psychiatric nursing and the care of the carers of the mentally ill at home, the comments of Brenton (1985) are pertinent. She stated:

> 'The informal deliverers of ''community care'' have saved the state a great deal of money, but the costs to *them* of this primary care are never included in the economic equations. ''Supporting the supporters'' has never been an instinctive goal of the statutory social services. More often than not, they have tended to ration their resources . . . their intervention delayed until the inevitable but initially preventable crisis has made more organised and expensive forms of care mandatory.'

This quotation accurately describes the situation as it exists in relation to the carers and the community psychiatric nursing services studied here. I would argue that no one professional can possibly have the solution to 'supporting the supporters' and caring for the mentally ill. Future research and service provision must be aimed at looking at the contributions of all workers with the mentally ill, including the 'informal' carers.

Appendix I

CONSENT FORM FOR MEDICAL STAFF AT WEST HOSPITAL

I am willing to give permission to LINDA POLLOCK to gain access to the case-notes and CPN records of:

1. ....

2. ....

3. ....

4. ....

5. ....

6. ....

7. ....

8. ....

9. ....

10. ....

I understand these individuals will be visited, interviewed and asked to complete a questionnaire within the next three months. I agree to this approach being made and will inform the researcher if I wish approval to be withdrawn. I also see no reason why an approach should not be made to the carer of these individuals.

.... Consultant's signature

.... Date

Appendix II

CONSENT FORM FOR PATIENTS INVOLVED IN THE STUDY AT
WEST HOSPITAL

I ....

....

(Insert name and address) hereby declare that:

a.   I know what I am being asked to do (for fuller details, see attached
sheet).

b.   An explanation has been given to me of any possible risks that
might occur.

c.   Having taken into consideration these factors, I agreed to
participate in this research project.

(Signed) ....   Date ....

I have a telephone, and also agree to being contacted by telephone if
necessary.

.... (Sign your initials if you agree)

Telephone number: .... Suitable time to 'phone ....

Appendix III

Pilot work with the tape-recorder allowed me to develop a check-list of activities which ensured that the taping of interviews in the main study was uneventful.

Power source

Using batteries
The machine I used had a red light which indicated whether or not the battery had been charged; half way through the first interview the battery failed and the tape stopped. To avoid this pitfall, I decided to recharge the batteries routinely before each interview (for several hours). If there was a choice, however, I used the mains lead.

Using the mains
I had to have an adaptor for round and square plug sockets; this was especially relevant as I was recording in different locations.

The interview room

Before meeting the subject to be interviewed, time needed to be spent in assessing the environment in which the interview was taking place. This included finding out where the mains switches were and ensuring that there was a table nearby for the tape-recorder; preferably this was at a good height to catch the voices of both questioner and respondent. Another important point was to organise the seating to facilitate relaxed conversation. This pre-interview organisation of furniture allowed the interview time to be used maximally for the research purpose and also avoided unnecessary upheaval.

Positioning of the tape-recorder

Recording was affected by the positioning of the tape-recorder and whether or not the respondent smoked and/or spoke clearly. Accurate positioning needed to be checked by testing recording during the first five minutes; this time was spent chatting about the day's work, and served the additional purpose of relaxing the interviewee.

Cassette-tapes

It was preferable to use known brands of tapes. In cheaper tapes, the notches at the back often failed to make contact and did not record (this was remedied by putting a piece of sellotape over the back notch to facilitate contact). It was always better to be confident that the taping was proceeding and I preferred to buy the more expensive tapes. A spare tape should always be taken to each interview in case of a fault occurring in one tape or an interview being lengthy.

Appendix IV

ORDER OF SYSTEMATIC PRESENTATION OF ELEMENT TRIADS

3	10	13
6	7	8
9	12	2
4	1	15
11	14	5
8	6	12
3	11	4
10	2	5
7	1	13
15	14	9
14	4	6
8	15	12
1	10	3
7	13	2
5	9	11

The presentation was calculated using random number tables and each element was used three times.

Appendix V

THE ELEMENTS USED IN THE TWO MAIN STUDY AREAS

Element Number	East Hospital	West Hospital
1	Lithium patient	GP referral
2	Depot patient	Depot patient
3	Other medication patient	HV referral
4	Consultant referral	Consultant referral
5	At-risk patient	At-risk patient
6	Depressive patient	Depressive patient
7	GP referral	Crisis calls
8	Requested visit	Home-assessment visit
9	Demented patient	Demented patient
10	Inpatient contact	Anxiety management
11	Physically ill	Social visit
12	Outpatient	SW referral
13	New referral	New referral
14	Chronic: actively involved in treatment, likely to change	
15	Chronic: not actively involved in treatment, not likely to change	

Appendix VI

ACTUAL CONSTRUCTS PRODUCED BY EACH NURSE, SORTED
UNDER HEADINGS OF THE CONTENT ANALYSIS

Home situation

Frank: Has practical support at home – lives on own
Lives in owner-occupied house – does not
Has family support – does not
Family has pathology – has not
Has people to stay with him – lives alone
Relatives are patients – are not
Has immediate family – does not
Has children – does not

Bert: Relatives know of illness – do not
Is hell to live with for relatives – liked as is
Lives with family – lives by self
Has small family – has widespread family
Is looked after by relative – is looked after by self
Is put in child's position, family speaks for him – is not
Relatives keep CPN informed – do not
Accepts help from family – does not

Adam: Has somebody at home – lives on own
Has child who isn't 'right' – does not
Has children – does not
Has tried to return to parental home – has not
Lives on own – does not
Has distant support – support lives locally
Support elusive as far as CPNs are concerned – easy access to relative
CPN contact with relatives is limited – is not

Hamish: Relative will contact CPN if problems – will not
Has support at home – lives alone
Family needs help and support – does not

Eddie: Gets on with person lives with – does not
Has responsibilities for looking after a family – has not
House sparse – house comfortable and clean
Is in sheltered housing – is not, has responsibilities

Kevin: Work with relatives – do not
Has support – has none at all

Home situation leaves a lot to be desired – stable household
Relationships are a difficulty – throwback from past

Lester: Has a stable background – does not
Has reasonable relationships at home – does not have stable relationships at home
Has got spouse involvement – has not
Has understanding and co-operative relatives – has not

Ivan: Family is supportive – is not
Lives alone – has family around
Lives alone – has relatives nearby
Is socially isolated – family is close by
Is influenced by mother – is not
Mother has control – has not
House is well kept – lives in appalling circumstances
Has children – has not

Graham: Is dependent emotionally on relatives – is not
Lives with relatives – lives alone
Has past problems with family which require support – does not need support with family
Relatives have problems, patient actively helps – does not
Has support at home – lives alone
Has family contact and support – does not
Has home help – does not
Has close family ties – does not

Colin: Is isolated – has family support
Family has had experience of caring – family has no experience of caring, find it difficult to cope
Family is in constant attendance – spends most of day by self
Is strain from time to time – is continual strain on family
Is strain on family – is not
Lives alone – does not
Is protected, lives in sheltered housing – is not
Lives alone – lives with family
Lives by self – lives with relatives

Dick: Has family support – has outside support
Has family at home – lives alone
Has social services support at home – has none
Has immediate family – has outside support
Lives alone – lives with family
Has immediate family – does not
Lives in council house – lives in sheltered housing
Lives upstairs – lives in flat
Lives with immediate family – lives alone

Has easy access to amenities – has not
Has phone – has not
Is at risk due to hearing loss – is not

Jock: Lives on own – lives with mother
Lives on own – lives with daughter
Is isolated – has family around
Has support of husband – does not

Illness

Frank: Neurotic overtones – psychotic
Is affective component to illness – is not
Has psychotic illness – has not
Has physical illness – has not
Has affective disturbance – has not
Has psychotic illness – has problems of everyday living
Is physically fit – is not

Bert: Is responding to excess anxiety – has psychiatric illness
Has physical illness – has not
Has periods of paranoid illness – has not
Has insight into illness – has not

Adam: Has physical illness – has not
Has schizophrenic illness – does not
Has mood swings – does not
Is together 'up top' – is mentally deteriorating
Is physically well – is not

Hamish: Has schizophrenic illness – has not
Is hypomanic – is not
Has good memory – is demented
Is 'together' – has memory blanks

Eddie: Is hysterical – is not
Is manic depressive – is not
Has physical problems – has not
Is suicide risk – is not
Diagnosis is decided – diagnosis is uncertain
Has temporal lobe epilepsy – has not
Is demented – is not

Graham: Threatens suicide, reacts histrionically to problems – does not
Has insight into present illness and situation – has not
Has psychotic illness – does not
No dementia – has dementia
Is suicidal – is not

Colin: Demented – is not
Organic – functional

Demented – functional
Has arthritis – has none
Had depression – has not had depression
Has grief reaction – has not
Demented – no memory impairment
Is sad within self – is happy within self

Dick: Is demented – is not
Has physical illness – has not
Has delusions and hallucinations – has not

Ivan: Has been on tranquillisers – has not
Has been addicted to tranquillisers – has not
Was addicted to medication – was never addicted
Is phobic – is not
Is agoraphobic – is not
Has panic attacks – has behavioural problems
Is anxious – is not
Understands what is happening to him – does not
Understands the illness – does not think there is anything
wrong
Is aware of what should be doing – lacks insight
Has been psychotic – has not
Is depressive – is not
Is suicidal – is not

Jock: Is psychotic – is confused

Kevin: Schizophrenic – anxiety state
Vague referral – specific referral
Diagnosis vague – diagnosis specific

Lester: Has a diagnosis – primarily a social problem
Is psychotic – is much more the social situation
Primarily had a diagnosis – primarily a social problem
Was diagnosed as ill – would not see self as such
Was diagnosed as psychiatric – was not
Was diagnosed as psychiatrically ill – was not

Treatment (a)

Bert: Has treatable disorder – has not
Responds quickly to intervention and help – does not
Is interested in continuing to be treated – 'cavalier'
attitude to mental illness
Is reluctant to have CPN – is happy to have CPN
Is unable to look after treatment if ill – is able to look after
treatment, can contact CPN
Is actively involved in treatment – is not

Hamish: Is regular attender – is not

            Is stuck in position has been in – is deteriorating

Graham: Is keen to come to day centre – is not
Has responded well to treatment – is still delusional
Is drain on day centre resources – is not
Has residual paranoid ideas – does not
Has responded to medication – has residual illness
Listens to what staff say – does not

Colin: Is confused at day centre – is not
Is dependent on day centre – is not
Enjoys day centre – does not

Dick: Unwilling to talk readily – gives information freely

Lester: Visits are beneficial – are not
Has benefited from CPN intervention – has not
CPN service is helping – is not

Ivan: Is resistive to suggestions – agrees in principle
Is resistive to suggestions – is responsive to suggestions
Is resistive to treatment – is co-operative

Jock: Has taken a lot of getting to know – has not

Kevin: Has poor prognosis – will never hear from again

Treatment (b)

Frank: Has been in hospital – has not

Bert: Has never been in hospital – has
Has been certified in past – has never been certified
Attends day centre – does not

Adam: Has had fair amount of psychiatric input – situational crisis

Hamish: Is outpatient – is inpatient
Has been in hospital – never
Has managed to keep out of hospital – has not

Eddie: Comes to number seven for treatment – does not
Is outpatient – is inpatient

Graham: Is in hospital – is not
Has required home visits – has not

Colin: Has been inpatient – has not
Needs to talk to solve problems – does not

Dick: Attends day centre – does not

Lester: Is GP referral – is not
Was referred by a psychiatrist – was not
Has been seen by psychiatrist – has not
Has had admissions – has not
Has been admitted to hospital – has not
Has ongoing supportive visits – has not

Has supportive visits – is offered active therapy
Is involved in active treatment – is not
Has long-term support visits – has passed on
Treatment became ongoing counselling – referred to other agencies
Needs long-term commitment from CPNs – does not
Is candidate for group therapy – is not
I have been involved in inactive work with him – I have not

Ivan: Attends anxiety management group – does not
Has had short stays in hospital – has not
Is working with relaxation tapes – is not
Would benefit from day care – would not
Comes to social club – does not

Jock: Has had various admissions to mental hospital – has not
Has had a lot of admissions to hospital – has not
Has the service that he requires – has not
Needs watching – does not
I go in and see how getting on – requires weekly injection
Needs counselling – is anxiety management case
Needs regular visiting – comes to group
Patient needs talking – mother needs talking
Patient needs support – relative needs support
Needs reassurance – does not

Kevin: I work on my own – I work with psychologist
I work by myself – I work with another professional
Is short term – will be difficult to discharge

Medication

Frank: Is on psychotropic medication – is not
Should be on medication – should not
Is on lithium – is not

Bert: Is on lithium – is not

Adam: Is unreliable in terms of medication – is reliable
Is on long term medication – is not
Is on injection – is not

Hamish: Is on lithium – is not
Has been on medication for years – has not

Eddie: Is on i.m. – is not

Graham: Is on lithium – is not
Is keen to take depot – is not
Is on depot – is not
Takes medication regularly – does not
Is on oral medication – is not

Is poor pill taker – is not
Has no difficulty with tablets – has difficulty

Colin: Has on-going psychiatric illness – is stabilised on medication

Dick: Is on psychotropic medication – is not

Ivan: Is on depot injections – is not

Kevin: Is on drugs – target is to come off drugs

Jock: Is on depot – is on oral medication
Is on depot – is not
Is on depot – I visit socially
Needs watching – looks after medication by self

Time orientation

Bert: Has always been something going on – is recent illness
Has long history – is short, recent illness
Has been suicidal in past – has not
Has recently been ill – has been stable for many years

Adam: Has lengthy experience of psychiatric care – contact with psychiatric care is recent
Will need supervision for long time – will be well soon
Is long-term patient – future unsure
Will be around for a while for CPNs – will not

Hamish: Is chronic – is a support patient
Has recent history of hospitalisation – has not
Has been here for past year – is chronic
Is chronic patient – is acute
Has been recently attending – has been for some time

Eddie: Is chronic – is not

Graham: Has long history of illness – is recent referral
Contact will be reduced in time – will always need support

Dick: Has long history – has short history

Kevin: First referral – known to service
In future, will have continued hospitalisations – will never

Lester: Has easily identified history – has not
Has psychotic background – has not
Will pop up again – is working things out

Ivan: Will not be on the books for long – is neurotic

Jock: Has been on the go for years – is recent contact
Is chronic – is GP referral

Social interaction

Frank: Enjoys going out – does not
Has social outlets – does not
Has interests – does not
Relies on public transport – has a car
Drives – does not

Bert: Has lot of people around him – has not
Difficult personality to get along with – is not
Gives information freely about background – does not
Goes out a lot – is socially inactive
Is outgoing – has never been 'life and soul'
Has hobbies – does not have interests outside self

Hamish: Is vocal – is quiet
Is social – is not
Will tell you if he has problems – needs probing

Eddie: Can be verbally aggressive to the nurses – is not

Graham: Is socially isolated – is outgoing
Is socially active – is isolated
Is sociable – is withdrawn socially

Colin: Joins in company – does not
Joins in socially – does not
Is deaf – is not

Dick: Is housebound – is fully ambulant
Is housebound – is capable of going out by self
Has mobility problems – is fully ambulant
Is deaf – is not

Lester: Has problems fitting into the community – does not

Ivan: Is socially isolated – is not
Is socially isolated – goes out and about
Has no-one – has friends to go out with

Work and money

Frank: Has job – does not
Is of employable age – is OAP
Works – does not

Bert: Is financed by self – is supported by another
Is financially well off – is not
Is retired – is working
Manages money – is financially subsidised
Is in debt – is not

Adam: Is in long term treatment – will hopefully go back to work

Eddie: Is unemployed – works

Is housewife – is not
Works full-time – does not

Graham: Finances are a discomfort – are not
Is long-term candidate for day care – hope will get a job
Is apt at handling money – is not
Can handle finances – cannot cope
Is keen to get to work – is not
Can budget – cannot
Has difficulty with money – has not

Ivan: Is unemployed – has a job
Is working – is not

Jock: Is comfortably off – has money worries

Self-sufficiency

Bert: Appears to run life OK – does not
Likes to run life for self – draws on helping agencies

Eddie: Needs bribing to have a bath – does not
Looks black – looks clean

Graham: Lacks personal hygiene – does not
Needs baths – does not
Is at risk in community – is not
Is realistic about life – is not

Colin: Needs reminding to do daily activities – can cope on own
Expects as much as possible to be done by family – is independent
Copes with everyday living – does not
Is preoccupied with past – is not
Can cope with everyday living – cannot cope with minor crisis

Dick: Is continent – is not

Ivan: Is dependent – lives a normal life
Is resistive to doing anything on own – is not

Jock: Has adjusted to retirement – has not

Lester: Is dependent – is not
Is keen on being in sick role – is not
Is mature – is not

Personal facts

Frank: Male – female
Young – pensioner

Bert: Working class – upper class

Eddie: Male – female

Graham: Smokes – does not
Normal intellect – average IQ

Colin: Working class – middle class

Dick: Male – female

Adam: Young – old

Ivan: Bright – borderline
Intelligent – slow

Self-reference

Frank: Irritates me – I warm to him/her
Lives in same place I do – does not

Hamish: I know well – I do not
I have known for some time – I am getting to know

Eddie: I know well – I do not know well

Ivan: I feel I am getting somewhere – I have given up
He is working at improving – I do not see improvement

Value judgement

Frank: Is manipulative – Is honest/open
Acts how feels – says how feels
Is hostile and dependent on professionals – is not
Is self-centred – puts others first
Is overweight – is skinny
Is nice basic person – is upper class
Is impulsive – is not
Seeks professional advice ad nauseam – does not

Eddie: Personality nice when well – is neurotic
Can be touchy and aggressive – is not
Is fat and healthy – gets emaciated

Graham: Is pre-occupied with illness – is not
Is sexually disinhibited – is not

Colin: Is restricted by religion – is not

Ivan: Is manipulative – is not
Is amenable – is not, is a lot of hard work
Is easy to communicate with – is not
Is attention seeking – is not

Problems isolated

Frank: Has sexual problems – does not
Has money problems – does not

Has drink problems – does not
Has physical problems – does not

Adam: Has drink problem – does not

Hamish Has weight problem – does not

Graham Has psychopathic problems – does not
Has problems with verbal communication – does not
Has overt behavioural problems – does not
Has identifiable problems – does not
Has organic cerebral problem – does not
Has personality problems – does not

Ivan: Has family problems – does not

Kevin Has problems with relatives – does not
Has relationship problems – has problems coping

Lester: Is a social problem – is not
Has real social problems – does not
Main involvement is to help cope with problems – is not
Has long-term problems – has new problems
Reasons for problems are obvious – are not

References

Adams R N and Preiss J J (eds.) *Human Organisation Research*. Illinois: Dorsey Press.

Age Concern (1984) *Some Facts About the Elderly in Scotland*. Edinburgh: Age Concern.

Aggleton P and Chalmers H (1986) *Nursing Models and the Nursing Process*. London: Macmillan Educational.

Ainsworth D and Jolley D (1978) The community nurse in a developing psychogeriatric service. *Nursing Times*, **74**(21): 873–874.

Allsop N (1980) *An Exploration of Infant Teachers' Explanations of Reading Difficulty*. MSc thesis, Edinburgh University.

Altschul A (1972a) A study of a multidisciplinary approach to treatment in the community with particular emphasis on the nursing role. Unpublished report, Edinburgh University.

Altschul A (1972b) *Patient–Nurse Interaction: A Study of Interaction Patterns in Acute Psychiatric Wards*. Edinburgh: Churchill Livingstone.

Altschul A (1972c) A study of the value of a multidisciplinary approach to treatment in the community with particular emphasis on the nursing role. Unpublished report, Edinburgh University.

Altschul A (1973) A multidisciplinary approach to psychiatric nursing. *Nursing Times*, **69**(15): 20–24.

Anderson D (1972) Working with the family doctor – a programme for mental health. *British Medical Journal*, **4**: 781–784.

Arie T H D (1972) In *Approaches to Action*, McLachlan G (ed.). Oxford: Oxford University Press, for the Nuffield Hospitals Trust.

Ashton J P C (1978) Community care in psychiatry – is it a myth? *Community Health*, **19**(4): 211–215.

Audit Commission (1986) *Making a Reality of Community Care*. London: HMSO.

Baker A A (1968) Psychiatric nursing in the community. In *The treatment of Mental Disorders in the Community*, Daniel G R and Freeman H L (eds). London: Ballière Tindall and Cassell.

Balfour-Sclare A (1971) The district nurse and community mental health. *Nursing Times*, **67**(35): 1080–1082.

Bannister D and Mair J M M (1968) *The Evaluation of Personal Constructs*. London: Academic Press.

Bannister D, Salmon P and Leiberman D M (1964) Diagnosis–treatment relationships in psychiatry. *British Journal of Psychiatry*, **110**: 726–732.

Banton R, Clifford P, Frosh S, Lousada J and Rosenthall J (1985) *The Politics of Mental Health*. Oxford: Macmillan.

Barker A and Black S (1971) An experiment in integrated psychogeriatric care. *Nursing Times*, **67**(45): 1395–1399.

Barker C (1977) A community psychiatric service. *Nursing Times,* **73**(28): 1075 – 1079.

Barker P (1986) *Assessment in Psychiatric Nursing.* London: Croom Helm.

Barker P and Fraser D (eds) (1985) *The Nurse as Therapist. A Behavioural Model.* London: Croom Helm.

Barrowclough C and Fleming I (1986) *Goal Planning with Elderly People. Making Plans to Meet Individual Needs. A Manual of Instruction.* Manchester: Manchester University Press.

Barrowclough C and Tarrier N (1984) Psychosocial interventions with families and their effects on the course of schizophrenia: a review. *Psychological Medicine,* **14**: 629 – 642.

Barton R (1959) *Institutional Neurosis.* Bristol: John Wright and Son.

Barton R and Lazersfeld P F (1969) Functions of a qualitative analysis in social research. In *Issues in Participant Observation,* McCall G J and Simmons J L. Massachusetts: Addison Wesley.

Baxter Y (1984) Conference report. *Community Psychiatric Nursing Journal,* **14**(3): 11.

Bayley M (1973) *Mental Handicap and Community Care.* London: Routledge and Kegan Paul.

Beail N (1985) *Repertory Grid Technique and Personal Constructs. Applications in Clinical and Educational Settings.* London: Croom Helm.

Beard P G (1980) Community psychiatric nursing–a challenging role. *Nursing Focus,* **1**(8): 306 – 307.

Bebbington P, Hurry J, Tennant C, Sturt E and Wing J K (1980) Epidemiology of mental disorders in Camberwell. *Psychological Medicine,* **10**: 185.

Becker H (1963) *Outsider: Studies in the Sociology of Deviance.* New York: The Free Press.

Becker H S and Geer B G (1960) The analysis of qualitative field data. In *Human Organisation Research,* Adams R N and Preiss J J (eds). Illinois: Dorsey Press.

Bellak L (1964) *Community Psychiatry and Community Mental Health.* New York: Grune and Stratton.

Berelson B (1952) *Content Analysis.* Illinois: Free Press.

Blaxter M (1976) *The Meaning of Disability: A Sociological Study of Impairment.* London: Heinemann.

Blenkner M (1950) Obstacles to evaluative research in casework, part 1. *Social Casework,* **31**: 54 – 60.

Bloch D (1975) Evaluation of nursing care in terms of process and outcome: issues in research and quality assurance. *Nursing Research,* **24** (4): 256 – 263.

Bloch S and Chodoff P (eds) (1981) *Psychiatric Ethics.* Oxford: Oxford University Press.

Blum H (1970) In *Qualitative Methodology: Firsthand Involvement with the Social World,* Filstead W J (ed.). Chicago: Markham Publishing.

Brennan P J (1981) A family close to crisis. *Nursing Times,* **77**(32): 1390 – 1392.

Brenton M (1985) *The Voluntary Sector in British Social Services.* New York: Longman.

British Medical Journal Editorial (1967) Future of mental hospitals. *British Medical Journal,* **ii** : 781.

Brook P and Cooper B (1975) Community mental health care: primary team and specialist services. *Journal of Royal College of General Practitioners*, **25**: 93–110.

Brooker C (1984a) The differences between community psychiatric nurses and behaviour therapists. Paper presented at the Kings Fund Conference, London.

Brooker C (1984b) Some problems associated with the measurement of community psychiatric nurse intervention. *Journal of Advanced Nursing*, **9**: 165–174.

Brooker C (1985a) *The 1985 National Community Psychiatric Nursing Survey Update: Implications of the Findings for the Evolution of a Survey Methodology*. MSc Thesis, London, City University.

Brooker C (1985b) Two psychiatric entities. *Nursing Mirror*, **160**(2): 35–36.

Brooking J (1986) *Psychiatric Nursing Research*. London: John Wiley and Sons.

Brough R (1980) Community psychiatric nurses' caseloads – how many? *Community Psychiatric Nurses Association Journal*, **1**(2): 12–13.

Brough R (1982) The community psychiatric nursing service at Prestwich Hospital. *Nursing Times*, **78**(19): 784–788.

Brown D and Pedder J (1979) *Introduction to Psychotherapy*. London: Tavistock Publications.

Brown G W (1973) Some thoughts on grounded theory. *Sociology*, **7**: 1–16.

Brown G W and Harris T (1978) *Social Origins of Depression: A Study of Psychiatric Disorder in Britain*. London: Tavistock.

Brown G W, Birley J L T, Wing J K (1972) Influence of family life on the course of schizophrenic disorders: a replication. *British Journal of Psychiatry*, **121**: 248–258.

Brown G W, Carstairs G M and Topping G (1958) The post hospital adjustment of chronic mental patients. *Lancet*, **ii**: 685–689.

Brown G W, Bone M, Dallison B and Wing J K (1966) *Schizophrenia and Social Care: a Comparative Follow-up Study of 339 Schizophrenic Patients*. London: Oxford University Press.

Brown G W, Monk E M, Carstairs G M and Wing J K (1962) Influence of family life on the course of schizophrenic illness. *British Journal of Preventative Social Medicine*, **16**: 55–68.

Brown P (ed.) (1985a) *Mental Health Care and Social Policy*. London: Routledge and Kegan Paul.

Brown P (1985b) *The Transfer of Care: Psychiatric Deinstitutionalisation and its Aftermath*. London: Routledge and Kegan Paul.

Burgess A W (1981) *Psychiatric Nursing in Hospital and Community*, 3rd edn. New Jersey: Prentice Hall.

Burgess A W (1985) *Psychiatric Nursing in Hospital and Community*, 5th edn. New Jersey: Prentice Hall.

Butterworth A and Skidmore D (1981) *Caring for the Mentally Ill in the Community*. London: Croom Helm.

Campbell D T and Stanley J C (1963) *Experimental and Quasi-Experimental Designs for Research*. Chicago: Rand McNally.

CANO (1975) *Review of Nursing Manpower Problems in Mental and in*

Deficiency Fields. Manpower Working Party Resources (Unpublished) Report. Edinburgh: Scottish Home and Health Department.

Caplan G (1964) *Principles of Preventive Psychiatry*. New York: Basic Books.

Carr P J, Butterworth C A and Hodges B E (1980) *Community Psychiatric Nursing: Caring for the Mentally Ill and Handicapped in the Community*. Edinburgh: Churchill Livingstone.

Cherniss C (1980) *Staff Burnout: Job Stress in the Human Services*. London: Sage.

Chenitz W C and Swanson J M (1986) *From Practice to Grounded Theory. Qualitative Research in Nursing*. California: Addison Wesley.

Chinn P L and Jacobs M K (1983) *Theory and Nursing*. St Louis: C V Mosby.

Clare A and Thompson S (1981) *Let's Talk about Me: A Critical Examination of the New Psychotherapies*. London: BBC.

Clarke M G (1980) Psychiatric liaison with the health visitor. *Health Trends*, **12**(4): 98–100.

Clarke P J (1982) Scotland's Mental Welfare Commission: a watchdog without any teeth. *Mindout*, Jan: 15–16.

Cochrane A L (1971) *Effectiveness and Efficiency: Random Reflections on Health Services*. London: Nuffield Provincial Hospital Trust.

Cohen D (1978) Psychiatry at home. *New Society*, March 2nd: 486–487.

Cohen S A (1981) Patient education: a review of the literature. *Journal of Advanced Nursing*, **6**: 11–16.

Community Psychiatric Nurses Association (1981) *The CPNA National Survey*. Bristol: CPNA.

Community Psychiatric Nurses Association (1983) *Mandatory Training of Community Psychiatric Nurses: Collated Comments of the Membership*. Bristol: CPNA.

Community Psychiatric Nurses Association (1985a) Regional roundup. *Community Psychiatric Nursing Journal*, **15**(6): 41.

Community Psychiatric Nurses Association (1985b) *The 1985 CPNA National Survey Update*. Bristol: CPNA.

Community Psychiatric Nurses Association (1985c) (Various examples) *Community Psychiatric Nursing Journal*, **5**(2): 3–4.

Community Psychiatric Nurses Association (1985d) *The Clinical Nursing Responsibilities of the Community Psychiatric Nurse*. Bristol: CPNA.

Cooper B, Harwin B G, Depla C and Shepherd M (1975) Mental health care in the community – an evaluative study. *Psychological Medicine*, **5**: 372–380.

Cormack D (1976) *Psychiatric Nursing Observed: a Descriptive Study of the Work of the Charge Nurse in Acute Admission Wards*. London: Royal College of Nursing.

Cormack D (1983) *Psychiatric Nursing Described*. Edinburgh: Churchill Livingstone.

Corrigan J and Soni D S (1977) Community psychiatric nursing: an appraisal of its impact on community psychiatry in Manchester, England. *Journal of Advanced Nursing*, **2**: 347–354.

Coverdale P R (1980) Community patterns of contact. *Nursing Times*, **76** (24): 1061–1062.

Craig R J S (1978) *Psychiatric Day Care Facilities with Particular Reference to Rosslynlee Hospital*. MPhil thesis, Edinburgh University.

Creer C and Wing J K (1974) *Schizophrenia in the Home.* Surbiton, Surrey: National Schizophrenia Fellowship.

Creer C, Sturt E and Wykes T (1982) The role of the relatives. In: Long term community care: experience in a London borough, Wing J K (ed). *Psychological Medicine,* Monograph Supplement 2.

Cronbach L J (1950) Further evidence on response sets and test design. *Educational Psychology Measurement,* **10**: 3–31.

Cumming E and Cumming J (1957) *Closed Ranks – An Experiment in Mental Health Education.* Cambridge, Massachusetts: Harvard University Press.

Davis B D (1984) A repertory grid study of formal and informal aspects of student nurse training. PhD thesis, London University.

Denham J (1972) Community psychiatry and the health service – now or never. *Public Health,* **86**: 53–56.

Denzin N K (1970) *The Research Act in Sociology.* Borough Green: Butterworth.

Department of Health and Social Security (1971) *Better Services for the Mentally Handicapped.* Cmnd 4683. London: HMSO.

Department of Health and Social Security (1974) *Report of the Enquiry into South Ockendon Hospital.* London: HMSO.

Department of Health and Social Security (1975) *Better Services for the Mentally Ill.* Cmnd 6233. London: HMSO.

Department of Health and Social Security (1976) *Priorities for the Health and Personal Social Services in England.* London: HMSO.

Department of Health and Social Security (1977) *The Way Forward.* London: HMSO.

Department of Health and Social Security (1979) *Royal Commission on the National Health Service* (The Merrison Report). Cmnd 7615. London: HMSO.

Department of Health and Social Security (1981a) *Care in Action.* London: HMSO.

Department of Health and Social Security (1981b) *Care in the Community.* London: HMSO.

Department of Health and Social Security (1981c) Letter from CNO DHSS. CNO(81)1D.

Department of Health and Social Security (1983) *Report of an Enquiry into the Management of the Health Service to the Secretary of State.* London: HMSO.

Department of Health and Social Security (1984) *Health Services Information* (The Korner Report). 5th Report to the Secretary of State. London: HMSO.

Department of Health for Scotland (1962) *Hospital Plan for Scotland.* Cmnd 1602. Edinburgh: HMSO.

Devlin R (1984) CPNs conference – a non-stop success. *Nursing Times, Community Outlook,* **80**(24): 207.

Devin R (1985) Training for the front line. *Nursing Times,* **81** (20): 19–20.

Dexter G and Morrall P (1987) All dressed up and nowhere to go: implications for the future of CPN education. *Community Psychiatric Nursing Journal,* 7(4): 11–15.

Diers D (1979) *Research in Nursing Practice.* New York: J B Lippincott.

Dimmock S (1985a) Big Business and the NHS. *Nursing Times,* **81**(5): 29–31.

Dimmock S (1985b) The attributes of excellence. *Nursing Times,* **81**(4): 28–30.

Dimmock S (1985c) What role for nurses? *Nursing Times,* **81**(8): 30–31.

Ditton L (1984) *Student Nurse Placement within the Community Psychiatric Nursing Team.* Unpublished paper, Hampstead District.

Donabedian A (1966) Evaluating the quality of medical care. *The Millbank Memorial Fund Quarterly,* **44**(3), part 2: 166–206.

Donabedian A (1983) Quality assessment and monitoring. *Evaluation and the Health Professionals,* **6**(3): 363–375.

Donnelly G (1977a) A day in the life of a community psychiatric nurse. *Nursing Mirror,* **114**(11): 38.

Donnelly G (1977b) Relationships: the social worker and the community psychiatric nurse. *Nursing Mirror,* **145**(12): 39–40.

Downie R S and Telfer E (1980) *Caring and Curing. A Philosophy of Medicine and Social Work.* London: Methuen.

Downie R S, Loudfoot E M and Telfer E (1974) *Education and Personal Relationships.* London: Methuen.

Driver E (1976) *Assessment of the Demand for a Community Psychiatric Nursing Service in Chester.* Monograph No 1. Manchester: Manchester Polytechnic.

Drucker N (1986) Lost in the haar: a critique of mental health in focus. *Scottish Government Yearbook,* pp.70–92. Edinburgh: SHHD.

Drucker N (1987) *Creating Community Mental Health Services in Scotland,* Volumes 1 and 2. Edinburgh: Scottish Association for Mental Health.

Duck S (1973) *Personal Relationships and Personal Constructs.* London: John Wiley and Sons.

Dunnell K and Dobbs J (1982) *Nurses Working in the Community: A Survey Carried Out on Behalf of the DHSS in England and Wales in 1980.* London: HMSO.

Eastwood B (1983) Care in the community. *Nursing Mirror,* **156**(2): 46.

Elliot-Cannon C (1981) Do the mentally handicapped need specialist community nursing care? *Nursing Times,* **77**(20): 77–80.

Epting F R, Suchman D I, and Nickson C J (1971) An evaluation of elicitation procedures for personal constructs. *British Journal of Psychology,* **62**(4): 513–517.

Equal Opportunities Commission (1980) *The Experience of Caring for Elderly and Handicapped Dependents: A Survey Report.* Manchester: EOC.

Equal Opportunities Commission (1982a) *Who Cares for the Carers? Opportunities for the Elderly and Handicapped.* Manchester: EOC.

Equal Opportunities Commission (1982b) *Caring for the Elderly and Handicapped: Community Care Policies and Women's Lives.* Manchester: EOC.

Equal Opportunities Commission (1984) *Carers and Services: A Comparison of Men and Women Caring for Dependent Elderly People.* Manchester: EOC.

Fadden I R, Bebbington P E and Kuipers L (1987) The burden of care: the impact of functional psychiatric illness on the patient's family. *British Journal of Psychiatry,* **150**: 285–292.

Fagbadegun R (1985) Management of neurosis. *Community Psychiatric Nursing Journal*, **15**(1): 24–25.

Falloon I, Boyd J L, McGill C W, Razani J, Moss H B and Gilderman A (1982) Family management in the prevention of exacerbations of schizophrenia. A controlled study. *New England Journal of Medicine*, **306**: 1437–1440.

Falloon R R H, Boyd J L and McGill C W (1984) *Family Care of Schizophrenia*. London: The Guilford Press.

Fawcett J (1984) *Analysis and Evaluation of Conceptual Models in Nursing*. Philadelphia: F A Davies.

Fenton F R, Tessier L, Struening E L, Smith F A and Benoit C (1982) *Home and Hospital Psychiatric Treatment*. London: Croom Helm.

Field P and Morse J (1985) *Nursing Research. The Application of Qualitative Approaches*. London: Croom Helm.

Fisch R, Weakland J H and Segal L (1982) *The Tactics of Change. Doing Therapy Briefly*. London: Jossey-Bass.

Fransella F and Bannister D (1977) *A Manual for Repertory Grid Technique*. London: Academic Press.

Freeman H E and Simmons O (1958) Mental patients in the community: family settings and performance levels. *American Sociological Review,* **23** (2): 147–154.

Freidson E (1970) *Profession of Medicine: A Study of the Sociology of Applied Knowledge*. New York: Dodd, Mead and Co.

Gardiner J (1981) Women, recession and the Tories. *Marxism Today*, **25** (3).

Gibbons J S, Horn S H, Powel J M and Gobbons J L (1984) Schizophrenic patients and their families. A survey in a psychiatric service based on a DGH unit. *British Journal of Psychiatry*, **144**: 70–77.

Gilhooly M L M (1984) The impact of care-giving on care-givers: factors associated with the psychological well-being of people supporting a dementing relative in the community. *British Journal of Medical Psychology*, **57**: 35–54.

Glaser B G and Strauss A (1967) *The Discovery of Grounded Theory: Strategies for Qualitative Research*. New York: Aldine.

Goddard H (1955) *The Work of the Mental Nurse*. Manchester: Manchester University Press.

Goddard H A (1958) *Principles of Administration Applied to Nursing Service*. Public Health Papers no. 41. Geneva: WHO.

Goffman E (1961) *Asylums: Essays on the Social Situation of Mental Patients and Other Patients*. New York: Doubleday.

Goffman E (1963) *Stigma: Notes on the Management of Spoiled Identity*. Harmondsworth: Penguin Books.

Goffman E (1964) *Behaviour in Public Places*. New York: The Free Press.

Goldberg D (1978) *The General Health Questionnaire*. Windsor: NFER.

Goldberg D and Huxley P (1980) *Mental Illness in the Community: the Pathway to Psychiatric Care*. London: Tavistock.

Gouldner A W (1959) Organizational analysis. In *Sociology Today: Problems and Prospects*, Merton R K, Broom L and Cottrell L S (eds). New York: Basic Books.

Grad J and Sainsbury P (1963) Mental illness and the family. *Lancet*, **i**: 544–547.

Grad J and Sainsbury P (1968) The effects that patients have on their families in a community care and a control psychiatric service. *British Journal of Psychiatry*, **114**: 265 – 278.

Greene J (1968) The psychiatric nurse in the community nursing service. *International Journal of Nursing Studies*, **5**: 175 – 183.

Griffith J H and Mangen S P (1980) Community psychiatric nursing – a literature review. *International Journal of Nursing Studies*, **17**: 197 – 210.

Habenstein R W and Christ E A (1955) *Professionalizers, Traditionalizers and Utilizers – An Interpretative Study of the Work of the General Duty Nurses in a Non-metropolitan Central Missouri General Hospital*. Columbia: University of Missouri Press.

Hadley R and Hatch S (1982) *Social Welfare and the Failure of the State: Centralised Social Services and Participatory Alternatives*. London: Allen and Unwin.

Haque G (1973) Psychosocial nursing in the community. *Nursing Times*, **69**(2): 51 – 53.

Harker P, Leopoldt H and Robinson J R (1976) Attaching community psychiatric nurses in general practice. *Journal of Royal College of General Practitioners*, **26**: 666 – 671.

Harrison B (1984) The community psychiatric nurse and the elderly – a manager's view. *Nursing Times*, **80**(39): 59.

Hawks D (1975) Community care: analysis of assumptions. *British Journal of Psychiatry*, **127**: 276 – 285.

Haywood S and Alaszewski S (1980) *Crisis in the Health Service*. London: Croom Helm.

Hazelden J (1981) *Exploring the Views of Four Guidance Teachers and Five Truants in a Scottish Secondary School*. MSc thesis, Edinburgh University.

Henderson B (1982) *A Study of the Frequency of Visits and Length of Involvement by Community Psychiatric Nurses at Winwick Hospital*. Dissertation for CPN course, Manchester Polytechnic.

Henderson J, Levin B and Cheyne E (1973) Role of a psychiatric nurse in a domiciliary treatment service. *Nursing Times*, **69**(41): 1334 – 1335.

Herz M I, Endicott J, Spitzer R L and Mesnikoff A (1971) Day versus in patient hospitalization : a controlled study. *American Journal of Psychiatry*, **127**: 1371 – 1382.

Higgins P (1984) Mental health education. *Nursing Mirror*, **159**(19): 28 – 29.

Hinkle D (1965) *The Change of Personal Constructs from the Viewpoint of a Theory of Implications*. Unpublished PhD thesis, Ohio State University.

Hoenig J (1974) The schizophrenic at home. *Acta Psychiatrica Scandinavia*, **50**: 297 – 308.

Hoenig J and Hamilton M W (1965) Extra-mural care of psychiatric patients. *Lancet*, **i**: 1322 – 1325.

Hoenig J and Hamilton M W (1967) The burden on the household in an extra-mural psychiatric service. In *New Aspects of the Mental Health Services*, Freeman H L and Farndale H L, (eds.), pp.612 – 635. London: Pergamon Press.

Hoenig J and Hamilton M W (1969) *The Desegregation of the Mentally Ill*. New York: Routledge and Kegan Paul.

Holloway R (1984) One step beyond. *Nursing Times*, **80**(8): 44 – 49.

Hooley J, Orley J and Teasdale J (1986) Levels of expressed emotion and relapse in depressed patients. *British Journal of Psychiatry*, **148**: 642–647.

Hughes D (1981) *Lay Assessment of Clinical Seriousness: Practical Decision-making by Non-medical Staff in a Hospital Casualty Department.* Unpublished PhD thesis, University of Wales.

Hume C and Pullen I (1986) *Rehabilitation in Psychiatry. An Introductory Handbook.* Edinburgh: Churchill Livingstone.

Hunt A (1978) *The Elderly at Home.* London: HMSO.

Hunter P (1974) Community psychiatric nursing in Britain: an historical review. *International Journal of Nursing Studies*, **11**: 223–233.

Hunter P (1978) *Schizophrenia and Community Psychiatric Nursing.* Surbiton, Surrey: The National Schizophrenia Fellowship.

Hunter P (1980) Social work and community psychiatric nursing – a review. *International Journal of Nursing Studies*, **17**: 131–139.

Hyman H, Wright C R and Hopkins T. (1962) *Applications of Methods of Evaluation: Four Studies of the Encampment for Citizenship.* Berkeley: University of California Press.

Illich I (1976) *Limits to Medicine. Medical Nemesis: The Expropriation of Health.* Harmondsworth: Penguin.

Illsley R (1980) *Professional or Public Health? Sociology in Health and Medicine.* London: The Nuffield Provincial Hospitals Trust.

Ingham J G (1965) A method of observing symptoms and attitudes. *British Journal of Social and Clinical Psychology*, **4**: 131–40.

James G (1961) Planning and evaluation of health programs. In *Administration of Community Health Services*, Confrey E A (ed.), pp. 114–134. Chicago: International City Managers Association.

Jeevendrampillai V (1982) Coming out of long stay. *Nursing Times*, **78** (18): 766–767.

Jeffery R (1979) Normal rubbish: deviant patients in casualty departments. *Sociology of Health and Illness*, **1**(1): 90–107.

John A (1961) *A Study of the Psychiatric Nurse.* Edinburgh: Churchill Livingstone.

Jones K and Poletti A (1985) Understanding the Italian experience. *British Journal of Psychiatry*, **146**: 341–347.

Judkins M (1976) *Introspective Dialogue Technique.* Unpublished manuscript. London: Royal Free Hospital.

Kalkman M (1974) The psychiatric nurse – historical development of role. In *New Dimensions in Mental Health Psychiatric Nursing*, Kalkman M and Davis A (eds), pp. 3–26. New York: McGraw Hill.

Kasper S (1962) Measurement of adjustment in adolescents: an extension of personal construct theory and methodology. *Psychological Monograph*, **6**(76): 1–32.

Kelly G E (1955) *The Psychology of Personal Constructs.* New York: Norton.

Kelly G E (1963) *A Theory of Personality.* New York: Norton.

Kendell R E (1975) Defining diagnostic criteria for research purposes. In *Methods of Psychiatric Research*, Sainsbury P and Kreitman N (eds), 2nd edn., pp. 101–119. London: Oxford Medical Publications.

Kennedy P and Hird F (1980) Description and evaluation of a short stay admission ward. *British Journal of Psychiatry*, **136**: 205–215.

Khandwalla M (1985) A specialist community psychiatric nursing service. *Community Psychiatric Nursing Journal*, **15**(1): 20–22.

King S (1962) *Perceptions of Illness and Medical Practice*. New York: Russell Sage Foundation.

Kirkpatrick W J A (1967) The in-and-out nurse. Some thoughts on the role of community psychiatric nursing and preparation required. *International Journal of Nursing Studies*, **4**: 225–231.

Kratz C (1974) *Problems of Care of the Long Term in the Community with Particular Reference to Patients with Stroke*. PhD thesis, Manchester University.

Kratz C (1987) Training for a takeover. *Nursing Times*, **83**(21): 16–17.

Kreisman D E and Joy V D (1974) Family response to the mental illness of a relative: a review of the literature. *Schizophrenia Bulletin*, **10**: 34–57.

Kreitman N (1961) The reliability of psychiatric diagnosis. *Journal of Mental Science*, **107**(450): 876–886.

Kreitman N (1964) The patient's spouse. *British Journal of Psychiatry*, **110**: 159–173.

Kuipers L (1987) Depression and the family. In *Coping with Disorder in the Family*, Orford J (ed). London: Croom Helm.

Landfield A (1971) *Personal Construct Systems in Psychotherapy*. New York: Rand McNally.

Langsley D G, Flomenhaft K and Machotka P (1969) Follow-up evaluation of family crisis therapy. *American Journal of Orthopsychiatry*, **39**: 753–759.

Leff J, Kuipers L, Berkowitz R, and Sturgeon D (1985) A controlled trial of social intervention in the families of schizophrenic patients: two year follow-up. *British Journal of Psychiatry*, **146**: 594–600.

Leff J, Kuipers L, Berkowitz R, Eberlein-Vries R and Sturgeon D (1982) A controlled trial of social intervention in the families of schizophrenic patients. *British Journal of Psychiatry*, **141**: 121–134.

Leff J P and Vaughn C E (1980) The interaction of life events and relatives' expressed emotion in relapse of schizophrenia and depressive neurosis. *British Journal of Psychiatry*, **136**: 146–153.

Leff J P and Vaughn C E (1981) The role of maintenance therapy and relatives' expressed emotion in schizophrenia: a two year follow-up. *British Journal of Psychiatry*, **139**: 102–104.

Leopoldt H (1973) Psychiatric community nursing. *Health and Social Services Journal*, **83**(4324): 489–490.

Leopoldt H (1974) The role of the psychiatric community nurse in the therapeutic team. *Nursing Mirror*, **138**(5): 70–72.

Leopoldt H (1975) GP attachment and psychiatric domiciliary nursing. *Nursing Mirror*, **140**(7): 82–84.

Leopoldt H (1979a) Community psychiatric nursing – 1. *Nursing Times Occasional Paper*, **75**(13): 53–56.

Leopoldt H (1979b) Community psychiatric nursing – 2. *Nursing Times Occasional Paper*, **75**(14): 57–59.

Leopoldt H and Hurn R (1973) Towards integration. *Nursing Mirror*, **136** (22): 38–42.

Leopoldt H, Hopkins H and Overall R (1974) A critical review of experimental nurse attachment scheme in Oxford. *Practice Team*, **3**(9): 2–6.

Leopoldt H, Robinson J R and Corea S (1975) Hospital based community psychiatric nursing in psychogeriatric care. *Nursing Mirror*, **141**(25): 54–56.

Lifshitz M (1974) Quality professionals. Does training make a difference? A personal construct theory. *British Journal of Social and Clinical Psychology*, **13**: 183–189.

Llewellyn E (1974) Community psychiatric nursing. *Midwife and Health Visitors Journal*, **10**(1): 7–9.

Lofland J and Lofland L (1984) *Analyzing Social Settings. A Guide to Qualitative Observation and Analysis*, 2nd edn. California: Wadsworth.

Lonsdale S, Flowers J and Saunders B (1980) *Long Term Psychiatric Patients: A Study in Community Care*. London: Personal Social Services Council.

Luker K (1982) *Evaluating Health Visiting Practice*. London: Royal College of Nursing.

McBrien M (1985) Paper presented at the Psychiatric Nurses Association Conference, Edinburgh.

McCall G and Simmons J L (1969) *Issues in Participant Observation: A Text and Reader*. Massachusetts: Addison Wesley.

McCreadie R G, Wilson O and Burton L L (1983) The Scottish survey of 'new Chronic' inpatients. *Psychiatry*, **143**: 564–571.

MacDonald D J (1972) Psychiatric nursing in the community. *Nursing Times*, **68**(3): 80–83.

McIlwaine H (1980) *The Nursing of Female Neurotic Patients in Psychiatric Units of General Hospitals*. PhD thesis, Manchester University.

MacKay J (1985) Reply of John MacKay to question by Malcolm Bruce on community psychiatric nursing, House of Commons, Jan 29th.

McKechnie A, Philip A and Ramage J (1981) Psychiatric services in primary care: specialised or not? *Journal of Royal College of General Practitioners*, **31**: 611–614.

McKendrick D (1980) *Statistical Returns: An Examination of Quantitative Methods in Use to Record the Activities of Community Psychiatric Nurses and Community Psychiatric Nursing Teams*. Research monograph no. 43. Manchester: Manchester Polytechnic.

McKendrick D (1981a) Statistical returns in community psychiatric nursing. *Nursing Times* Occasional Paper, **77**(26): 101–104.

McKendrick D (1981b) Statistical returns in community psychiatric nursing. *Nursing Times* Occasional Paper. **77**(27): 108.

Mair J M M (1966) Prediction of grid scores. *British Journal of Psychology*, **57**: 187–192.

Maisey M (1975) Hospital based psychiatric nursing in the community. *Nursing Times*, **71**(9): 354–355.

Manchester J (1984) Nurse therapists and community psychiatric nurses. Paper presented at the Kings Fund Conference, London.

Mangen S P and Griffith J H (1982a) Community psychiatric nursing services in Britain: the need for policy and planning. *International Journal of Nursing Studies*, **19**(3): 157–166.

Mangen S P and Griffith J H (1982b) Patient satisfaction with community psychiatric nursing: prospective controlled trial. *Journal of Advanced Nursing*, **7**: 477–482.

Marais R A (1976) Community psychiatric nursing – an alternative to hospitalisation. *Nursing Times*, **72**(44): 1708–1717.

Marks I (1985) Controlled trial of psychiatric nurse therapists in primary care. *British Medical Journal*, **290**: 1181–1184.

Martin J P (1984) *Hospitals in Trouble*. Oxford: Basil Blackwell.

May A R (1965a) Psychiatry within the general hospital. *Nursing Mirror*, **121** (3157): 427–432.

May A R (1965b) Psychiatry within the general hospital. *Nursing Mirror*, **121** (3158): 461–465.

May A R and Moore S (1963) The mental nurse in the community. *Lancet*, i: 213–214.

May D and Kelly M P (1982) Chancers, pests and poor wee souls: problems of legitimation in psychiatric nursing. *Sociology of Health and Illness*, **4**(3): 279–301.

Mayer J E and Timms N (1980) *The Client Speaks, Working Class Impressions of Casework*. London: Routledge and Kegan Paul.

Mechanic D (1968) *Medical Sociology*. London: Collier Macmillan.

Melia K M (1981) *Student Nurses' Accounts of their Work and Training, a Qualitative Analysis*. PhD thesis, Edinburgh University.

Mental Welfare Commission (1981) *Does the Patient Come First?* Edinburgh: HMSO.

Mental Welfare Commission (1986) *Mental Welfare Commission for Scotland Report for 1985*. Edinburgh: HMSO.

Menzies I E P (1960) A case study in the functioning of social systems as a defence against anxiety. *Human Relations*, **13**: 95–121.

Miller J B (1976) *Toward a New Psychology of Women*. Boston: Beacon Press.

Mills E (1962) *Living with Mental Illness: A Study in East London*. London: Routledge and Kegan Paul.

Milverton R (1985) Institutional neurosis amongst clients living in the parental home. *Community Psychiatric Nursing Journal*, **15**(1): 11–13.

Ministry of Health (1962) *A Hospital Plan for England and Wales*. Cmnd 1604. London: HMSO.

Ministry of Health Central Health Services Council (1968) *Psychiatric Nursing: Today and Tomorrow*. London: HMSO.

Mitchell A (1973) What is your label? *Mind and Mental Health Magazine*, 1973: 32–35.

Moore J (1982) No place like home? *Nursing Times*, **78**(9): 353.

Mulhall D J (1971) *On Trends of Subjective Experience*. Unpublished dissertation for the British Psychological Society Diploma in Clinical Psychology.

Mulhall D J (1976) Systematic self-assessment by PQRST. *Psychological Medicine*, **6**: 591–597.

Mulhall D J (1978) *Manual for Personal Questionnaire Rapid Scaling Technique*. Windsor: NFER.

Murray J E (1974) Patient participation in determining psychiatric treatment. *Nursing Research*, **23**(4): 325–333.

Nickerson A (1972) Psychiatric community nurses in Edinburgh. *Nursing Times*, **68**(10): 289–291.

Nie N H (1975) *SPSS Users Guide*. Illinois: McGraw Hill.

Nie N H (1983) *SPSSX Users Guide*. Illinois: McGraw Hill

Nightingale F (1859) *Notes on Nursing*. Harrisson and Sons. Reprinted 1980 by Churchill Livingstone, Edinburgh.

Norris M (1981) Problems in the analysis of qualitative data – suggested solutions. *Sociology*, **15**(3): 337 – 351.

Oldfield S (1983) *The Counselling Relationship*. London: Routledge and Kegan Paul.

Oppenheim A and Eemen B (1955) *The Function and Training of Mental Nurses*. London: Chapman and Hall.

Oppenheim A N (1983) *Questionnaire Design and Attitude Measurement*. 9th edn. London: Heinemann.

Orford J (ed) (1987) *Coping with Disorder in the Family*. London: Croom Helm.

Page R (1984) *Stigma: Concepts in Social Policy*. London: Routledge and Kegan Paul.

Pai S and Kapur R L (1982) Impact of treatment intervention on the relationship between dimensions of clinical psychopathology, social dysfunction and burden on the family of psychiatric patients. *Psychological Medicine*, **12**: 651 – 658.

Pai S and Nagarajaiah H (1982) Treatment of schizophrenic patients in their homes through a visiting nurse – some issues in nurse training. *International Journal of Nursing Studies*, **19**(3): 167 – 172.

Parnell J W (1974) Psychiatric nursing in the community. *Queen's Nursing Journal*, **27**(2): 36 – 38.

Parnell J W (1978) *Community Psychiatric Nursing: A Descriptive Study*. London: Queen's Nursing Institute.

Parsons T (1958) Definitions of health and illness in light of American values and social structure. In *Patients, Physicians and Illness*, Jaco E (ed). New York: The Free Press.

Paykel E S and Griffith J H (1983) *Community Psychiatric Nursing for Neurotic Patients: The Springfield Controlled Trial*. London: Royal College of Nursing.

Paykel E S, Mangen S P, Griffith J H and Burns T F (1982) Community psychiatric nursing for neurotic patients – a controlled trial. *British Journal of Psychiatry*, **140**: 573 – 581.

Pearsall M (1965) Participant observation as role and method in behavioural research. *Nursing Research*, **14**(1): 37 – 41.

Penfold P S and Walker G A (1983) *Women and the Psychiatric Paradox*. Milton Keynes: Open University Press.

Peplau H E (1952) *Interpersonal Relations in Nursing*. New York: Putnam.

Peplau H E (1960) Talking with patients. *American Journal of Nursing*, **60**: 964 – 966.

Peplau H E (1962) Interpersonal techniques: the crux of psychiatric nursing. *American Journal of Nursing*, **62**: 50 – 54.

Persaud T (1985) The general student in the community. *Community Psychiatric Nursing Journal*, **5**(1): 6 – 10.

Personal Social Services Council London/Central Health Services Council (1979) *Collaboration in Community Care – A Discussion Document*. London: HMSO.

Pharaony N and Mills N (1976) *Attitudes of Other Agencies Towards*

Community Psychiatric Nurses. Research monograph no. 6. Manchester: Manchester Polytechnic.

Philip A E and McCulloch J W (1968) Personal construct theory and social. work practice. *British Journal of Social and Clinical Psychology*, **7**: 115 – 121.

Pilkington T (1973) Public and professional attitudes to mental handicap. *Public Health*, **87**: 61 – 66.

Platt S (1985) Measuring the burden of psychiatric illness on the family: an evaluation of some rating scales. *Psychological Medicine*, **15**: 383 – 393.

Platt S and Hirsch S (1981) The effects of brief hospitalization upon the psychiatric patient's household. *Acta Psychiatrica Scandinavica*, **64**: 199 – 216.

Platt S, Weyman A, Hirsch S and Hewitt S (1980) The social behaviour assessment schedule (SBAS): rationale, contents, scoring and reliability of a new interview schedule. *Social Psychiatry*, **15**: 43 – 55.

Politics of Health Group (Undated) Cuts and the National Health pamphlet no. 2 and Going private – the case against private medicine. In *The Politics of Nursing*. Salvage J, 1985. London: Heinemann Medical.

Pollock L C (1986a) An introduction to the use of repertory grid technique as a research method and clinical tool for psychiatric nurses. *Journal of Advanced Nursing*, **11**: 439 – 445.

Pollock L C (1986b) In *Rehabilitation in Psychiatry*, Hume C and Pullen I (eds). Edinburgh: Churchill Livingstone.

Pollock L C (1987) *Community Psychiatric Nursing Explained: An Analysis of the Views of Patients, Carers and Nurses*. PhD thesis, Edinburgh University.

Pollock L C (1988) The work of community psychiatric nursing. *Journal of Advanced Nursing*, **13**: 537 – 545.

Pope M L and Keen T R (1981) *Personal Construct Psychology and Education*. London: Academic Press.

Powell D (1982) *Learning to Relate – A Study of Student Psychiatric Nurses' Views of Preparation and Training*. London: Royal College of Nursing.

Power D (1976) *Extending the Community Psychiatric Nursing Service in Doncaster*. Monograph no. 8. Manchester: Manchester Polytechnic.

Psychiatric Nurses Association of Scotland (1986) *A Proposal for Change in RMN Training*. Dundee: PNAS.

Pullen I (1980) Decription of an extramural service for psychiatric emergencies. *Health Bulletin*, **38**: 163 – 166.

Pullen I and Gilbert M A (1979a) Crisis team turn chaos into relief. *Nursing Mirror*, **149**(14): 34 – 35.

Pullen I and Gilbert M A (1979b) When crisis hits the home. *Nursing Mirror*, **149**(13): 30 – 32.

Quine L (1981) Alone in the community. *New Society*, **56**: 435 – 436.

Raphael W (1972) *Patients and their Hospitals*. London: Kings Fund.

Ratna L (undated) In *Reassessing Community Care*, Malin N, 1987. London: Croom Helm.

Redman B K (1980) *The Process of Patient Teaching in Nursing*, 4th edn. St Louis: C V Mosby.

Reed J and Lomas G (eds) (1984). *Psychiatric Services in the Community*. London: Croom Helm.

Rees T P (1957) Back to moral treatment and community care. *Journal of Mental Science*, **103**: 303–313.

Reynolds B (1985) Issues arising from teaching interpersonal skills in psychiatric nurse training. In *Interpersonal Skills in Nursing*, Kagan C (ed), pp. 228–247. London: Croom Helm.

Rhodes M (1986) *Ethical Dilemmas in Social Work Practice*. London: Routledge and Kegan Paul.

Riehl J P and Roy C (eds) (1980) *Conceptual Models for Nursing Practice*. Norwalk: Appleton Century Crofts.

Ritson B (1977) Psychiatry and the community. *Contact*, **2**: 27–31.

Roberts L (1976) The community psychiatric nurse. *Nursing Times*, **72** (51): 2020–2021.

Rogers C R (1957) The necessity and sufficient conditions of therapeutic personality change. *Journal of Consulting Psychology*, **21**: 95–103.

Rosenhan D L (1973) On being sane in insane places. *Science*, **179**: 250–258.

Rosenthal R and Fode K L (1963) Psychology of the scientist: three experiments in experimenter bias. *Psychological Reports*, **12**: 491–511.

Rossi P H and Williams H (1972) *Evaluating Social Programs, Theory, Practice and Politics*. New York: New York Seminar Press.

Roth I (1976) *Social Perception*. Reader, Block 8, Course D305. Milton Keynes: Open University.

Rowe D (1971) An examination of a psychiatrist's predictions of a patient's constructs. *British Journal of Psychiatry*, **118**: 231–234.

Royal College of General Practitioners (1981) *Prevention of Psychiatric Disorders in General Practice*. London: Royal College of General Practitioners.

Royal College of Nursing (1981) *Towards Standards: Second Report of RCN Working Committee on Standards of Nursing Care in England and Wales*. London: Royal College of Nursing.

Royal College of Nursing (1982a) *Mandatory Training for Community Psychiatric Nurses – The Way Forward*. A joint statement from the Royal College of Nursing and the Community Psychiatric Nurses Association. London: Royal College of Nursing.

Royal College of Nursing (1982b) Seminar on advanced clinical roles, 8 – 9 March. London: Royal College of Nursing.

Royal College of Psychiatrists (1980) The role and responsibilities of the community psychiatric nurse. *Royal College of Psychiatrists Bulletin*, **9**.

Royal Commission on the Law Relating to Mental Illness and Mental Deficiency (1957) Cmnd 169. London: HMSO.

Royal Commission on the National Health Service (1979) Cmnd 7615. London: HMSO.

Rushforth D (1986) *An Evaluation of the Management of Deliberate Self Harm Employing the CPN as an Agent of Change*. MPhil thesis, Manchester Polytechnic.

Rutter M (1966) The reliability and validity of measures of family life and relationships in families containing a psychiatric patient. *Social Psychiatry*, **1**(1): 38–54.

Ryce S (1978) Psychiatric nursing from a health centre. *Nursing Mirror*, **147**(7): 35–36.

Salvage J (1985) *The Politics of Nursing*. London: Heinemann Medical.

Sarbin T R and Mancuso J C (1970) Failure of a moral enterprise, attitudes of the public towards mental illness. *Journal of Consulting and Clinical Psychology*, **33**: 159–175.

Scheff T J (1966) *Being Mentally Ill*. London: Weidenfeld and Nicholson.

Schwartz M S and Shockley E L (1956) *The Nurse and the Mental Patient*. London: John Wiley and Sons.

Scott W A (1962) Cognitive complexity and cognitive flexibility. *Sociometry*, **25**(1): 405–414.

Scottish Action on Dementia (1986a) *Dementia: Action on Training*. Edinburgh: Scottish Action on Dementia.

Scottish Action on Dementia (1986b) *A Dementia Studies Centre: A Strategy for the Development of Services for Dementia Sufferers and their Carers*. Edinburgh: Scottish Action on Dementia.

Scottish Association of Mental Health (1984) *Briefing Papers – Mental Health Matters*. Edinburgh: Scottish Action on Mental Health.

Scottish Home and Health Department (1976) *The Health Service in Scotland: The Way Ahead*. Edinburgh: HMSO.

Scottish Home and Health Department (1979a) *A Better Life: Report on Services for the Mentally Handicapped in Scotland*. Edinburgh: HMSO.

Scottish Home and Health Department (1979b) *Services for the Elderly with Mental Disability in Scotland (The Timbury Report)*. Edinburgh: HMSO.

Scottish Home and Health Department (1980a) *Changing Patterns of Care: Report on Services for the Elderly in Scotland*. Edinburgh: HMSO.

Scottish Home and Health Department (1980b) *SHAPE Report: Scottish Health Authorities Priorities for the Eighties*. Edinburgh: Scottish Home and Health Department.

Scottish Home and Health Department (1981) *Continuing Education for the Nursing Profession in Scotland*. Report of a working party on continuing education and professional development for nurses, midwives and health visitors. Edinburgh: Scottish Home and Health Department.

Scottish Home and Health Department (1983) *Health in Scotland 1982*. Edinburgh: HMSO.

Scottish Home and Health Department (1985) *Mental Health in Focus*. Edinburgh: HMSO.

Scottish Working Group (1984) *Community Care – Joint Planning and Support Finance Arrangements*. Edinburgh: Scottish Working Group.

Scottish Working Group (1985) *Community Care: Strategy for Action*. Edinburgh: Scottish Working Group.

Sencicle L (1981) Which way the CPN? *Community Psychiatric Nurses Association Journal*, **2**(1): 10–14.

Shanley E (1984) *Evaluation of Mental Nurses by their Patients and Charge Nurses*. PhD thesis, Edinburgh University.

Shapiro M B (1961) A method of measuring psychological changes specific to the individual psychiatric patient. *British Journal of Medical Psychology*, **34**: 151–155.

Sharpe D (1975) Role of the community psychiatric nurse. *Nursing Mirror*, **141**(16): 60–62.

Sharpe D (1980) Figures tell their own story. *Nursing Mirror*, **150** (2): 34–36.

Sharpe D (1982) GPs' views of community psychiatric nursing. *Nursing Times*, **78**(40): 1664–1666.

Shaw A (1977) CPN attachment in a group practice. *Nursing Times*, **73** (12): ix–xvi.

Shepherd M, Irving D and Davies G (1966) *Psychiatric Illness in General Practice*. London: Oxford University Press.

Shires J (1977) A travelling day hospital – an experiment in rural community care. *Social Work Today*, **8**(24): 16–18.

Shore A (1977) *An Objective Appraisal of the Existing Community Psychiatric Nursing Services in NW Region of NHS with a View to Making Recommendations for the Future Development of the Rochdale Service*. Monograph no. 19. Manchester: Manchester Polytechnic.

Shubachs A P W (1975) To repeat or not to repeat? Are frequently used constructs more important to the subjects? A study of the effect of allowing repetition of constructs in a repertory test. *British Journal of Medical Psychology*, **48**: 31–37.

Sieber S D (1976) *A Synopsis and Critique of Guidelines for Qualitative Analysis Contained in Selected Textbooks*. Unpublished paper. Project on social architecture in education. New York: Centre for Policy Research.

Siegel S (1956) *Nonparametric Statistics for the Behavioural Sciences*. London: McGraw Hill.

Simmons S and Brooker C (1986) *Community Psychiatric Nursing: A Social Perspective*. London: Heinemann.

Simms L M (1981) The grounded theory approach in nursing. *Nursing Research*, **30**(6): 356–359.

Singer M T and Wynne L C (1965) Thought disorder and family relations of schizophrenics, iv: Results and implications. *Archives of General Psychiatry*, **12**: 201–212.

Skidmore D and Friend W (1984a) CPNs need enrolled nurses. *Nursing Times, Community Outlook*, **80**(32): 299 – 301.

Skidmore D and Friend W (1984b) Muddling through. *Nursing Times*, **80** (19): 179–180.

Skidmore D and Friend W (1984c) Over to you. *Nursing Times, Community Outlook*, **80**(41): 369–371.

Skidmore D and Friend W (1984d) Should CPNs be in the primary health care team? *Nursing Times, Community Outlook*, **80**(38): 257–260.

Skidmore D and Friend W (1984e) Specialism or escapism. *Nursing Times, Community Outlook*, **80**(24): 203–205.

Skidmore D and Friend W (1984f) Student rethink needed. *Nursing Times, Community Outlook*, **80**(27): 257–260.

Sladden S (1977) *Psychiatric Community Nursing: A Study of a Working Situation*. PhD thesis, Edinburgh University.

Sladden S (1979) *Psychiatric Nursing in the Community: A Study of a Working Situation*. Edinburgh: Churchill Livingstone.

Slater P (1976) *Explorations of Interpersonal Space, Volume 1*. London: John Wiley and Sons.

Slater P (1978) *Dimensions of Interpersonal Space, Volume 2*. London: John Wiley and Sons.

Smith P and Kendall L M (1963) Retranslation of expectations: an approach to the construction of unambiguous anchors for rating scales. *Journal of Applied Psychology,* **47**: 149–155.

Social Services Committee (1985) *Community Care: Second Report to the House of Commons* (The Short Report). London: HMSO.

Spitzer R L, Gibbon M and Endicott J (1971) *Family Evaluation Form. Biometrics Research.* New York: New York State Department of Mental Hygiene.

Spradley J P (1980) *Participant Observation.* New York: Holt, Rinehart and Winston.

Stacey M (1969) The myth of community studies. *British Journal of Sociology,* no.20.

Stanfield I (1984) Weeding out the victims. *Nursing Times, Community Outlook,* **80**(27): 238–240.

Stevens B C (1972) Dependence of schizophrenic patients on elderly relatives. *Psychological Medicine,* **2**: 17–32.

Stewart V and Stewart A (1981) *Business Application of Repertory Grid.* London: McGraw Hill.

Stobie E and Hopkins D (1972a) Crisis intervention, 1 : a community psychiatric nurse in a rural area. *Nursing Times,* **68**(43): 165–168.

Stobie E and Hopkins D (1972b) Crisis intervention, 2. *Nursing Times,* **68**(43): 169–172.

Stockwell F (1972) *The Unpopular Patient.* London: Royal College of Nursing.

Strong P (1980) Doctors and dirty work: the case of alcoholism. *Sociology of Health and Illness,* **12**: 24–47.

Struening E and Guttentag M (1975) *Handbook of Evaluation Research.* Beverley Hills: Sage Publications.

Suchman E A (1967) *Evaluative Research.* New York: Russell Sage Foundation.

Sullivan H S (1953) *The Interpersonal Theory of Psychiatry.* New York: Norton.

Tarrier N and Barrowclough C (1986) Providing information to relatives about schizophrenia: some comments. *British Journal of Psychiatry,* **149**: 458–463.

Thomas L F and Harri-Augstein E S (1985) *Self-Organised Learning. Foundations of a Conversational Science for Psychology.* London: Routledge and Kegan Paul.

Thompson I E, Melia K M and Boyd K M (1983) *Nursing Ethics.* Edinburgh: Churchill Livingstone.

Timms N and Watson D (1978) *Philosophy in Social Work.* London: Routledge and Kegan Paul.

Tizard J A and Grad J (1961) *The Mentally Handicapped and their Families.* Maudsley Monograph no. 7. London: Oxford University Press.

Topliss I and Gould B (1981) *A Charter for the Disabled.* Oxford: Martin Robertson.

Tough H, Elliot P and Kingerlee P (1980) Surgery attached psychogeriatric nurses: an evaluation of psychiatric nurses in the primary care team. *Journal of the Royal College of General Practitioners,* **30**: 85–89.

Towell D (1975) *Understanding Psychiatric Nursing*. London: Royal College of Nursing.

Townsend P (1981) Elderly people with disabilities. In *Disability in Britain: A Manifesto of Rights*, Walker A and Townsend P (eds) pp.91–118. Oxford: Martin Robertson.

Townsend P and Davidson N (1982) *The Inequalities of Health*. Harmondsworth: Penguin.

Turner B A (1981) Some practical aspects of qualitative data analysis: one way of organising the cognitive processes associated with the generation of grounded theory. *Quality and Quantity*, **15**: 225–247.

Tyrell M (1975) *Using Numbers for Effective Health Service Management*. London: Heinemann Medical.

United Kingdom Central Council for Nurses, Midwives and Health Visitors (1984) *Code of Professional Conduct*. London: UKCC.

United Kingdom Central Council for Nurses, Midwives and Health Visitors (1985) *Project 2000: The Future Professional Practice of Nursing, Midwifery and Health Visiting*. London: UKCC.

Vaughn C E and Leff J P (1976a) Influence of family and social factors on the course of psychiatric illness – a comparison of schizophrenia and depressed neurotic patients. *British Journal of Psychiatry*, **129**: 125–137.

Vaughn C E and Leff J P (1976b) The measurement of expressed emotion in families of psychiatric patients. *British Journal of Social and Clinical Psychology*, **15**: 157–165.

Walker A (ed) (1982) *Community Care: The Family, the State and Social Policy*. Oxford: Basil Blackwell and Martin Robertson.

Walker A, Omerod P and Whitty L (1979) *Abandoning Social Priorities*. London: CPAG.

Warren J (1971) Long acting phenothiazine injections given by psychiatric nurses in the community. *Nursing Times* Occasional Paper, **67**(36): 141–143.

Washburn S, Vannicelli M, Longabaugh R and Scheff B J (1976) A controlled comparison of psychiatric day treatment and in-patient hospitalisation. *Journal of Consulting Psychology*, **44**: 665–675.

Waters M A and Northover J (1965) Rehabilitated long-stay schizophrenics in the community. *British Journal of Psychiatry*, **111**: 258–267.

Watson J P (1970) A measure of therapist–patient understanding. *British Journal of Psychiatry*, **117**: 319–321.

Weeks K and Greene J (1966) Nursing after care in psychiatry. *Nursing Times*, **65**(51): 1629.

Wertheimer A (1982) *Living for the Present*. Community Mental Health Enquiry Paper no. 9.

Wheatley V (1980a) Relative stress. *Community Care*, 22–23.

Wheatley V (1980b) *Supporters of Elderly Persons with a Dementing Illness Living in the Same Household*. MSc thesis, Surrey University.

White E G (1983) *'If it's Beyond me'* . . .: *Community Psychiatric Nurses in Relation to General Practice*. MSc thesis, Cranfield Institute.

White E G and Mangan J (1981) *Community Psychiatric Nursing – Roots to Branches*. Report to Chief Nursing Officer. Unpublished monograph, Hastings Health Authority.

Wilding P and George V (1984) *The Impact of Social Policy.* London: Routledge and Kegan Paul.

Willey R (1969) Nursing after care in psychiatry. *Nursing Times,* **65**(51): 1629.

Williamson F (1982) The nursing process in a community psychiatric nursing service. *Nursing Times* Occasional Paper, **78**(1): 1–3.

Williamson F, Little M and Lindsey W (1981) Two community psychiatric nursing services compared. *Nursing Times* Occasional Paper, **77**(27): 105–107.

Wilson E (1982) In *Community Care: The Family, the State and Social Policy,* Walker A (ed) pp.40–55. Oxford: Basil Blackwell and Martin Robertson.

Wilson-Barnett J (1983) *Nursing Research: Ten Studies in Patient Care.* Chichester: John Wiley and Sons.

Wing J K and Brown G W (1961) Social treatment of schizophrenia: a comparative survey of three mental hospitals. *Journal of Mental Science,* **107**: 862.

Wing J K and Brown G W (1970) *Institutionalisation and Schizophrenia.* London: Cambridge University Press.

Wiseman J (1981) Community nurses and health care recording. *Nursing Times* Occasional Paper, **77**(28): 109–112.

Wolfenden Committee Report (1978) *The Future of Voluntary Organisations.* London: Croom Helm.

World Health Organisation (1978) *Mental Disorders: Glossary and Guide to their Classification in Accordance with the Ninth Revision of the International Classification of Diseases.* Geneva: World Health Organisation.

Wright C (1955) Evaluating mass media campaigns. *International Social Science Bulletin,* **7**: 3.

Wright K J T (1970) Exploring the uniqueness of common complaints. *British Journal of Medical Psychology,* **43**: 221–232.

Yorke D M (1978) Repertory grids in educational research: some methodological considerations. *British Educational Research Journal,* **4**: 63–74.

Yura R and Walsh M B (1967) *The Nursing Process.* Norwalk: Appleton Century Crofts.

Zola I (1972) Medicine as an institution of social control. *Sociological Review,* **20**: 487–504.

The RCN Research Series

Background Information

The RCN Research Series was founded in 1971 by the DHSS and the RCN. The Series is published by a division of the RCN's subsidiary company, Scutari Projects (Scutari Press). Since the first publication ('A Family Visitor') in 1973, more than 50 monographs have been produced. The majority of authors are nurses, but suitable studies by non-nurse authors have been published. The Series, in its new, larger format, is now available through booksellers as well as through Scutari Projects.

The aim of the Series is to encourage the appreciation and dissemination of nursing research by making relevant studies available to the profession.

The Series has made an impact on nurse practitioners, educators and managers, and it has contributed to the promotion of nursing as a research-based profession. The Series is recognised both nationally and internationally.

The RCN, in accordance with its policy of promoting research appreciation and understanding among members of the profession, commends this Series for study, but the views expressed do not necessarily reflect RCN policy.

Individuals are invited to submit research reports to be considered for inclusion in the Series. In the first instance reports should be submitted to the Publisher (Scutari Press). Manuscripts can be submitted in the form of a Masters or Doctoral degree thesis. Research projects undertaken in partial fulfilment of a course or basic degree are not normally considered suitable. In any event, prospective authors are encouraged to send in research reports soon after completion so that the work is not out of date.

The RCN Librarian would be grateful to receive copies of Masters and Doctoral theses on nursing for the Steinberg Collection.